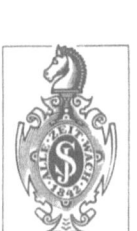

N. A. Romas · E. D. Vaughan (Eds.)

Alternate Methods in the Treatment of Benign Prostatic Hyperplasia

With 67 Figures and 26 Tables

Springer-Verlag
Berlin Heidelberg NewYork
London Paris Tokyo
Hong Kong Barcelona Budapest

Nicholas A. Romas, M.D.

Department of Urology, St. Luke's/Roosevelt Hospital Center, 428 West 59th Street, NewYork, NewYork 10019, USA

E. Darracott Vaughan, M.D.

New York Hospital-Cornell Medical Center, 525 East 68th Street, NewYork, NewYork 10021, USA

ISBN-13: 978-3-642-45725-8   e-ISBN-13: 978-3-642-45723-4
DOI: 10.1007/978-3-642-45723-4

Library of Congress Cataloging-in-Publication Data
Alternate methods in the treatment of benign prostatic hyperplasia. Nicholas A. Romas, E. Darracott Vaughan (eds.). p. cm. Includes bibliographical references and index.
ISBN-13: 978-3-642-45725-8
1. Prostate–Hypertrophy. I. Romas, Nicholas A., 1936-. II. Vaughan, E.D. [DNLM: 1. Prostatic Hypertrophy–therapy.

This work is subject to copyright. All rights are reserved, whether the whole or part of the material is concerned, specifically the rights of translation, reprinting, re-use of illustrations, recitation, broadcasting, reproduction on microfilms or in other ways, and storage in data banks. Duplication of this publication or parts thereof is only permitted under the provisions of the German Copyright Law of September 9, 1965, in its current version and a copyright fee must always be paid. Violations fall under the prosecution act of the German Copyright Law.

© Springer-Verlag Berlin Heidelberg 1993
Softcover reprint of the hardcover 1st edition 1993

The use of registered names, trademarks, etc. in this publication does not imply, even in the absence of a specific statement, that names are exempt from the relevant protective laws and regulations and therefore free for general use.

Product liability: The publisher can give no guarantee for information about drug dosage and application thereof contained in this book, in every individual case the respective user must check its accuracy by consulting other pharmaceutical literature.

Cover design: Erich Kirchner, Heidelberg
Typesetting: Laserwords, Madras
21/3020 5 4 3 2 1 0 Printed on acid-free paper

Contributors

Reginald Bruskewitz, M.D.
Department of Urology, Center of Health Sciences, University of Wisconsin-Madison, 600 Highland Avenue, Madison, Wisconsin 53792, USA

S. Larry Goldenberg, M.D., F.R.C.S.C.
Department of Urology, St. Paul's Hospital, University of British Columbia, Vancouver, British, Columbia V6Z 2A5, Canada

John T. Grayhack, M.D.
Department of Urology, Northwestern University Medical School, 303 East Chicago Avenue, Chicago, Illinois 60611, USA

Placido Grino, M.D.
Clinical Research-Endocrinology and Metabolism, Merck Sharp & Dohme Research Laboratories, P.O. Box 2000, Rahway, New Jersey 07065, USA

Harry A. Guess, M.D., Ph.D.
Epidemiology Department, Merck Sharp & Dohme Research Laboratories, West Point, Pennsylvania 19486-004, USA

Steven A. Kaplan, M.D.
College of Physicians and Surgeons, Columbia University, 630 West 168th Street, New York, New York 10032, USA

James M. Kozlowski, M.D.
Department of Urology, Northwestern University Medical School, 303 East Chicago Avenue, Chicago, Illinois 60611, USA

Chung Lee, Ph.D.
Department of Urology, Northwestern University Medical School, 303 East Chicago Avenue, Chicago, Illinois 60611, USA

Herbert Lepor, M.D.
Departments of Urology, Pharmacology and Toxicology, Medical College of Wisconsin, 9200 West Wisconsin Avenue, Milwaukee, Wisconsin 53226, USA

Franklin C. Lowe, M.D., M.P.H.
Department of Urology, St. Luke's/Roosevelt Hospital Center, 428 West 59th Street, New York, New York 10019, USA

Winston K. Mebust, M.D.
Section of Urology, University of Kansas Medical Center, 3901 Rainbow Boulevard, Kansas City, Kansas 66160-7390, USA

Aaron P. Perlmutter, M.D., Ph.D.
Department of Surgery, Division of Urology, The New York Hospital-Cornell Medical Center, 525 East 68th Street. New York, New York 10021, USA

Morton Riehmann, M.D.
Department of Urology, Center of Health Sciences, University of Wisconsin-Madison, 600 Highland Avenue, Madison, Wisconsin 53792, USA

Robert A. Roth, M.D.
Department of Urology, Lahey Clinic Medical Center, 41 Mall Road, Burlington, Massachusetts 01805, USA

Elizabeth Round, Ph.D.
Clinical Research-Endocrinology and Metabolism, Merck Sharp & Dohme Research Laboratories, P.O. Box 2000, Rahway, New Jersey 07065, USA

Nelson N. Stone, M.D.
Elmhurst Hospital Center, Mount Sinai School of Medicine, 79-01 Broadway, Elmhurst, New York 11373, USA

Elizabeth Stoner, M.S., M.D.
Clinical Research-Endocrinology and Metabolism, Merck Sharp & Dohme Research Laboratories, P.O. Box 2000, Rahway, New Jersey 07065, USA

Maryrose P. Sullivan, Ph.D.
Division of Urology, Veterans Administration Medical Center, Harvard Medical School, 1400 VFW Parkway, West Roxbury, Massachusetts 02132, USA

Alan, J. Wein, M.D.
Division of Urology, Hospital of the University of Pennsylvania, 3400 Spruce Street - 5 Silverstein, Philadelphia, Pennsylvania 19104, USA

Subbarao V. Yalla, M.D.
Division of Urology, Veterans Administration Medical Center, Harvard Medical School, 1400 FVW Parkway, West Roxbury, Massachusetts 02132, USA

Contents

Preface

In the field of Urology, no treatment of a particular disease has changed so markedly over a short period of time as it has for benign prostatic hyperplasia (BPH). Up to several years ago, patients with prostatism had two choices for treatment. The patient was either treated with a prostatectomy, or the operation was deferred until the patient became more symptomatic.

The present text attempts to summarize the main treatment options for BPH but realizes that the field is evolving so rapidly that it may well be outdated by the time of publication. The treatment options may be divided into minimally invasive or medical treatment of BPH. The minimally invasive methods include transurethral incision of the prostate, balloon dilatation of the prostate, prostate urethral prosthesis, prostate heat treatments, and laser prostatectomy. Medical management consists of alpha-adrenergic blockade, 5 alpha-reductase inhibitors, flutamide, and aromatase inhibitors.

Many important questions arise, but patient selection is perhaps foremost. Who should receive medical management? Will multiple drug therapy be an improvement over monotherapy? Who is most likely to benefit from one of the minimally invasive procedures and which one? Next, over what time period are these treatments effective? In short, will alternative treatment replace prostatectomy or simply defer it? Lastly, what approach will be most economical as medicine enters into a tighter cost containment era? These and other questions will hopefully be answered in the near future.

The editors are extremely grateful to the contributing authors for the high quality of their manuscripts. We thank the St. Luke's-Roosevelt Urology Residents Dr. Edward Stark, Dr. Stephen Trauzzi, Dr. Delbert Kwan, and Dr. Carlton Barnswell for their work on the index and Ms. Marilyn Carlin for her help in the coordination of the project.

N.A. Romas
E.D. Vaughan

Natural History of Benign Prostatic Hyperplasia

H.A.Guess

Introduction

The natural history of a disease refers to its evolution over time in the absence of treatment. While benign prostatic hyperplasia (BPH) is a common disorder in men over 50 years of age and accounts for 1.7 million physician office visits and nearly 400 000 prostatectomies annually in the United States, few natural history studies of BPH have been conducted (Barry 1990a, b). Many urologists have probably followed more untreated BPH patients in their own practices than have been described in all the natural history studies published in the urologic literature.

Much of the controversy concerning indications for treating BPH is traceable to a lack of quantitative information about BPH natural history and long-term outcomes of treatment. A recent review article on controversies about indications for transurethral resection of the prostate states the case for natural history information succinctly,

> "Most men with symptoms of benign prostatic hypertrophy are not predes-
> tined for obstructive uropathy or acute urinary retention. For most patients the
> decision to operate should be made by the patient after being fully informed.
> However, for patients to be truly informed we need additional information
> regarding the natural history of the disease, and we need clinical trials that
> provide more direct information on the outcomes of different treatments or
> treatment versus non-treatment." (Graversen et al. 1989)

At the World Health Organization International Consultation on BPH, in June 1991, the need for additional information on BPH natural history was again emphasized. Studying the onset and evolution of BPH in large numbers of men should help provide a better base of information for patients and their urologists to use in deciding on monitoring and intervention strategies.

This chapter provides an overview of the natural history of anatomically and clinically diagnosed BPH. Main results from published studies will be reviewed briefly, emphasizing recent findings. Finally, research in progress from two commu-nity-based BPH natural history studies will be mentioned. The latter studies are designed to determine the prevalence and progression of male urologic findings related to BPH through long-term follow-up of several thousand men randomly sampled from the general population of one community in Scotland and one in the United States. All of the work in this chapter pertains to untreated BPH.

Anatomic Prevalence and Progression

In one sense BPH is an anatomic diagnosis and it is in this sense that its origin and evolution have been most clearly described. McNeal showed that BPH nodules originate in a region of the prostate (transition zone and periurethral gland region) located near the proximal urethra and comprising about 2% of the total prostate mass and 5%–10% of the mass of glandular tissue (McNeal 1978, 1990). He identified three pathological processes involving: (1) nodule formation, (2) diffuse transition zone enlargement, and (3) nodule enlargement (McNeal 1978; Walsh 1992).

Berry further traced the anatomic progression of BPH using data from ten autopsy studies involving more than 1000 prostates (Berry et al. 1984). Prior to puberty the average prostate weight was 1.6 g. With the onset of puberty prostate weight increased rapidly, reaching about 20 g by age 21–30. This average weight was approximately maintained for all later decades in those prostates with no histologic evidence of BPH. By contrast, in the prostates with histologic evidence of BPH there was a gradual increase in average weight with increasing age. For men age 50 and older the rate of increase was roughly 0.6 g/year. However, the weight distribution of prostates which were histologically normal at autopsy showed considerable overlap with the weight distribution of prostates found to contain histological evidence of BPH. The mean weight of histologically normal prostates was 21 g with a standard deviation of 6 g and the mean weight of prostates with histological evidence of BPH was 33 g with a standard deviation of 16 g. Only 4% of the prostates in men over 70 years of age weighed more than 100 g. The highest reported prostate weight in BPH appears to be 1058 g, in a 55 year-old Caucasian man (Tolley et al. 1987).

Prostate growth rates based on autopsy studies must be interpreted with caution, since the growth rates are based on weights measured in different groups of people at different ages rather than on measurements in individual patients followed over time. Almost no data exists on serial prostate size measurements in individual patients followed over several years. In a Japanese study, Ohnishi followed 16 patients with periodic transrectal ultrasound measurements over 7 years and concluded that some patients had very rapid periods of prostate growth over a few years in the sixth decade, with little further change in prostate size (Ohnishi et al. 1987).

Clinical Prevalence

Much less is known about clinically diagnosed BPH than about anatomically diagnosed BPH. Widely accepted clinical diagnostic criteria for BPH do not exist (Barry 1990b). Some studies have defined BPH simply as prostate enlargement, as measured by manual rectal examination (Glynn et al. 1985), transrectal ultrasonography (Ohnishi et al. 1987; Watanabe et al. 1977), or autopsy (Randall 1931). However, manually determined prostate size is both poorly reproducible – as evidenced by a high degree of interobserver variability (Meyhoff and Hald 1978) – and inaccurate – as evidenced by poor agreement with prostate weights determined at surgery (Meyhoff et al. 1981). Prostate size as measured by transrectal ultrasonography has shown good agreement with surgically defined prostate size (Hricak et al. 1987), but the latter does not correlate with urodynamic measures of bladder outflow obstruction or with symptomatic improvement following prostatectomy and is only weakly correlated with obstructive urologic symptoms (Graversen et al. 1989; Jensen et al. 1983). Also, as discussed above, there is considerable overlap in the weight distributions of histologically normal prostates and prostates with histologic evidence of BPH. Hence diagnosing BPH clinically based on prostate size alone would be neither anatomically accurate nor relevant to the clinical problem of deciding whether a patient has a condition (bladder outflow obstruction caused by BPH) which a prostatectomy for BPH is likely to improve (Walsh 1986; Graversen et al. 1989).

To understand why prostate size correlates poorly with histologically diagnosed BPH or with bladder outflow obstruction due to BPH it suffices to consider where and how BPH develops. Because the expansile nodules of BPH originate in a highly localized periurethral region occupying less than about 2% of total prostate mass, it is possible for obstruction to occur without much increase in prostate size. Alternatively, diffuse enlargement of the transition zone may produce considerable increase in prostate size without much obstruction.

Different diagnostic criteria for BPH give rise to widely different prevalence estimates. In Figure 1 the first bar shows the prevalence of BPH defined in a Scottish community using a diagnostic criterion based on symptom score, urinary flow rate, and prostate size by transrectal ultrasound (Garraway et al. 1991). The second and third bars show the prevalence of BPH diagnosed by enlarged prostate on digital rectal examination in two United States populations: (1) men taking physical examinations to qualify for life-insurance (Lytton 1983) and (2) the Baltimore Longitudinal Study of Aging (BLSA), a long-term study of human aging conducted by the National Institute on Aging (Guess et al. 1990). These two age-specific prevalences are somewhat higher than that based on the clinical criteria shown in the first bar.

The fourth bar shows the prevalence of prostatism (BPH diagnosed clinically on the basis of a medical history and digital rectal examination) in the Baltimore Longitudinal Study of Aging. This is much higher than the prevalence of manually determined prostate enlargement in the same men (third bar) but shows surprisingly close agreement with histologic prevalence estimates of Berry et al. (1984), shown in the fifth bar. Although the close agreement between histologic BPH and prostatism in each of four decades may represent coincidence, it is also possible that histologic BPH may be more closely related to clinical prostatism than the large amount of individual variation might lead one to expect (Guess et al. 1990).

Whatever case definition is used, BPH is common among men over 50 years of age and it increases in prevalence with increasing age. Differences in age-specific

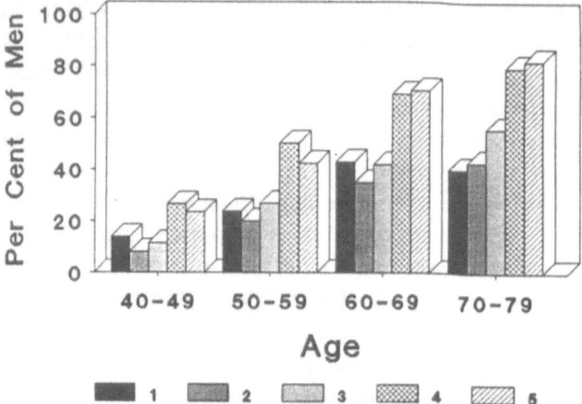

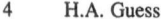

Fig. 1. Age-specific prevalence of benign prostatic hyperplasia. *1* Community prevalence in Bridge of Allan, Scotland based on a case definition using symptoms, prostate size, and urinary flow rates (*n* = 699) (Garraway et al. 1991); *2* clinical prevalence based on an enlarged prostate on manual rectal examination from a compilation of life insurance examinations (*n* = 6975) (Lytton 1983); *3, 4* clinical prevalence in the Baltimore Longitudinal Study of Aging (BLSA) (*n* = 1057) (Guess et al. 1990): *3* based on presence of an enlarged prostate on manual rectal examination, *4* based on history and physical examination; *5* prevalence of pathologically defined BPH from a compilation of five autopsy studies (*n* = 1075) (Berry et al. 1984)

prevalence between studies in which different BPH diagnostic criteria were used may be due either to different diagnostic criteria or to biological differences between the populations.

Clinical Progression

Follow-Up Studies of Untreated BPH Patients

Four main follow-up studies of untreated BPH patients have been conducted in England and the United States. Clarke used Boston hospital outpatient records to follow 93 men with BPH for an average period of 4 years (Clarke 1937). Spontaneous improvement was common, particularly among men with milder disease. During the follow-up period 29 (31%) of these patients had a prostatectomy.

Craigen conducted a follow-up study of 251 British men who had consulted their general practitioners for urologic symptoms (Craigen et al. 1969): 39 (16%) of these men were eventually found to have prostate cancer and were analyzed separately; 89 (42%) of the remaining 212 presented in acute urinary retention and eight additional men developed acute retention subsequently. Of the 115 remaining men in whom retention did not develop, 48 (42%) had a prostatectomy during the 7 year follow-up period. Nearly half of those who did not have a prostatectomy were free of symptoms at final follow-up 4–7 years after the initial visit.

Birkhoff followed an American population of 53 untreated BPH patients, of whom 26 were followed without treatment for 3 years (Birkhoff et al. 1976). Nine untreated men with BPH developed acute retention. Ball followed 107 British men with prostatism in whom prostatectomy was not initially indicated (Ball et al. 1981). During a follow-up period of up to 5 years only ten (9%) had a prostatectomy (two for acute retention and the other eight for worsening symptoms and low flow rates). The other 97 patients remained untreated. On 5 year follow-up 31 (32%) reported symptom improvement and 50 (52%) reported that their symptoms were the same. Urinary flow rates in the patients who eventually had surgery were lower than in those who did not, but the predictive value of flow rate measurements was not stated. Urinary flow measurements 5 years apart were available on 64 of the untreated BPH patients. The averages of the maximum flow rates at the beginning and end of the 5 year follow-up periods were 13.1 ml/s and 11.9 ml/s, representing an average decline of about 1.2 ml/s over 5 y, or about 0.2 ml/s per year. This rate, based on long-term follow-up of individual untreated BPH patients, is in agreement with the value of 2.1 ml/s per 10 years of age found in a study of normal men, in which the rate of decline was inferred from single measurements on men of different ages (Drach et al. 1979).

Together, these studies show that the clinical course of BPH varies greatly and that many BPH patients without clear indications for surgery improve without treatment. However, it is not possible to predict the course of individual patients. It would be difficult to know how to interpret more quantitative comparisons of these studies because of the small numbers of patients studied, differences in how the data were collected, lack of information about patient selection, and lack of information about completeness of follow-up. The annual incidence of acute urinary retention in these studies differed by more than a factor of ten, ranging from 0.4%. (based on two cases) to 6% (based on nine cases). One of the problems in judging the risks of not treating BPH has been the lack of reliable estimates of the risk of complications such as acute retention, chronic retention, bladder decompensation, hydronephrosis, or pyelonephritis (Graversen et al. 1989; Barry 1990a).

Information about BPH from Long-Term Studies of Human Aging

Since studies of untreated BPH patients start with symptomatic patients referred for urologic evaluation, they do not provide information on the prevalence of urologic symptoms in the community. Also, their applicability to the general male population or even to a primary care setting is limited by the selected nature of the patients. Because BPH has a gradual onset men will wait varying lengths of time before presenting for medical care. Thus, a study based on enrolling patients who have presented for medical care will miss early disease and cannot properly describe the natural history of BPH from its inception. To study BPH from its inception, it would be desirable to begin with a random sample of the general male population within the age range of interest who have never received treatment for BPH. These men could then be followed over time with periodic questionnaires and examinations to study the onset and evolution of BPH over time in a community setting. Such studies are both difficult and expensive to organize. Hence, as a first step in this direction, it makes sense to see what information on urologic conditions can be obtained from several ongoing epidemiologic studies of human aging in which populations of several thousand men have been followed for 20–30 years with periodic health questionnaires and physical examinations. Results from three such studies have been published to date.

In a prospective study of 2036 male volunteers (The Normative Aging Study) Glynn examined potential predictors of prostatectomy for BPH, while controlling for age (Glynn et al. 1985). *Decreased* risk of prostatectomy for BPH was associated with smoking. *Increased* risks of prostatectomy for BPH were associated with prior clinical diagnosis of enlarged prostate, Jewish religion, and lower socioeconomic status. Based on the incidence of prostatectomy in this study, it was calculated that about 29% of men who survive to age 80 can be expected to have had a prostatectomy for BPH.

Sidney reported results of a prospective study of 16 219 male members of the Kaiser Permanente Medical Care Program, a prepaid health care program that serves about one-quarter of the population of the San Francisco Bay Area in California (Sidney et al. 1991a). The men in this study were sampled from Kaiser enrollees without regard to urinary symptoms. They received multiphasic health examinations (including health questionnaires) during 1971–1972 and were followed until membership termination or the end of 1987. In multivariate analyses controlling for age, decreased risks of prostatectomy for BPH were associated with alcohol consumption of three or more drinks per day, smoking, obesity, and glucose intolerance. Increased risks of prostatectomy for BPH (controlling for age) were independently associated with a urine pH of 6 or more, a history of kidney or bladder infection, a history of tuberculosis, and several other factors that related to medical care history. In a separate analysis of urologic symptoms in relation to subsequent prostatectomy for BPH, the following urologic symptoms were independently predictive of prostatectomy (controlling for age): hesitancy, weak stream, painful urination, loss of bladder control, and nocturia.

The decreased risk of prostatectomy associated with high alcohol intake is consistent with autopsy studies showing cirrhosis (mainly alcoholic cirrhosis) to be negatively associated with histologically diagnosed BPH (Bennett et al. 1950; Frea et al. 1987; Robson 1966; Stumpf and Wilens 1953). An inhibitory effect of alcohol on BPH would be biologically plausible in view of known effects of alcohol (even without cirrhosis) on testosterone metabolism (Gordon et al. 1976). The finding that obesity is associated with decreased risk of prostatectomy could also have a hormonal basis. Some of the other associations identified may have to do more with fitness for surgery than with any etiologic effect on BPH. For example, the finding by both Glynn and Sidney, that smoking was associated with a decreased risk of prostatectomy for BPH, may reflect an association between smoking and pulmonary conditions that would be relative contraindications to elective surgery rather than any biological effect of smoking on BPH itself. In view of the large number of possible associations tested in these studies, all of these findings must be viewed as conjectures for further study rather than as established causal relationships.

Sidney also compared the age-specific incidence of surgery in white and black male enrollees in the Kaiser population (Sidney et al. 1991b). In this prepaid health plan enrollees or their employers pay a monthly fee that covers essentially all medical and surgical care. Hence rates of prostatectomy among Kaiser enrollees would not be expected to be influenced by differences in access to care or by patient income. The overall age-adjusted rates of prostatectomy for BPH were identical in the two racial groups, while the rate of prostate cancer was 80% higher in blacks than in whites. Thus, the well-known higher incidence of prostate cancer among blacks does not translate into a higher risk of surgically operated BPH. Blacks had a slightly higher incidence of prostatectomy for BPH than whites under age 65, while the reverse was true over age 65. A similar finding of a slight tendency for BPH to present earlier in blacks than in whites was found more than 50 years ago (D'Aunoy et al. 1939).

Arrighi analyzed data from the Baltimore Longitudinal Study of Aging (BLSA) involving 1057 men followed for up to 30 years with periodic general health questionnaries and physical examinations (Arrighi et al. 1990). Men with manually determined prostate enlargement and obstructive symptoms were several times more likely to require prostatectomy for BPH than men without these findings. Of 112 men with manually determined prostate enlargement plus the symptoms of weak stream and a sensation of incomplete emptying, 41 (37%) eventually had a prostatectomy for BPH. Of the remaining 945 only 69 (8%) came to prostatectomy for BPH. The symptom most highly predictive of prostatectomy was a weak stream. Thus prostatectomy for BPH was quite uncommon in men who did not have at least two obstructive symptoms, but only a minority of men with prostatism came to surgery for BPH. Figure 2 shows the progression of four urologic symptoms with increasing age in this population. The symptom of "weak stream" was present in about 25% of men in their mid-50s, this increased to nearly 50% for men in their mid-70s. While nocturia was even more prevalent in this population, it had no predictive relationship to subsequent prostatectomy for BPH.

Complications of BPH

The main sources of morbidity and mortality with BPH are renal failure, urologic infections leading to pyelonephritis and sometimes to sepsis, acute urinary retention, and mortality from complications of therapy (Birkhoff 1983). Quantitative epidemiologic information on the likelihood of these complications and on what risk factors may be most important is lacking (Barry 1990a, b).

Bacteriuria has been found in about 9% of men with BPH without urinary tract instrumentation, increasing to 15% with instrumentation (Andersen and Vejlsgaard 1980; Hasner 1962). Bladder calculi were found to be about eight times more prevalent at autopsy in men age 60 and over with BPH than in comparably aged men without BPH (3.4% vs 0.4%), while the prevalence of kidney and ureter stones was nearly identical (6.0% vs 5.7%) (Grosse 1990). Information on the frequency of renal impairment in BPH comes mainly from surveys of men undergoing prostatectomy for PPH and from surveys of hospital admissions for renal failure. Neither

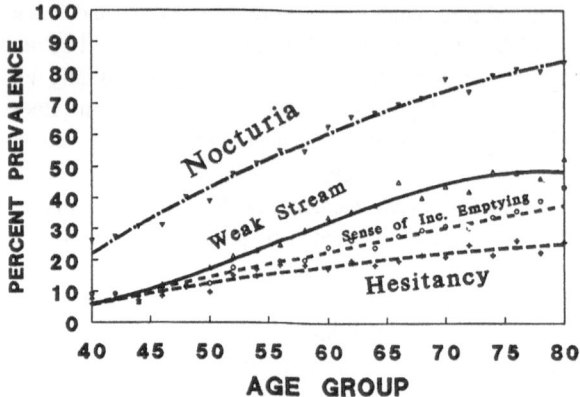

Fig. 2. Urologic symptoms in men according to the Baltimore Longitudinal Study of Aging

type of survey permits calculating incidence. Elevated plasma creatinines were found in 7% of men at the time of prostatectomy (Sacks et al. 1989) and upper urinary tract dilatation has been reported in 5% of men being investigated in-hospital for prostatism (Abrams et al. 1976). In a review of community-acquired acute renal failure presenting to the Boston VA Medical Center, 17% of the cases were due to urinary obstruction, of which 65% were considered to be caused by BPH (Kaufman et al. 1991). These results imply that BPH is responsible for an appreciable fraction of acute renal failure among older men and at least several percent of men coming to prostatectomy for BPH have evidence of clinically signif-icant renal impairment.

Estimates of the incidence of acute urinary retention among men with BPH are based on a few small studies. As discussed earlier, risk estimates from these studies vary widely (0.4%–6% per year). Acute urinary retention is unpredictable in onset and men who develop it do not tend to be among the most highly symptomatic (Birkhoff et al. 1976; Powell et al. 1980). There is some evidence to suggest that prostatic infarction may be a factor in the pathogenesis of some cases of acute urinary retention (Graversen et al. 1989; Spiro et al. 1974). While acute urinary retention is often the initial presenting complaint in men with BPH, it can also occur following nonurological surgery in men who do not have BPH (Andersen and Grant 1991).

Prostate Cancer Risk Among Men With BPH

The relationship between BPH and prostate cancer has been investigated in two conflicting studies (Armenian et al. 1974; Greenwood et al. 1974). The study which found a positive association has been criticized over the selection of controls and the lack of histologic confirmation of BPH (Franks 1974; Williams and Blackard 1974). Since the histologically distinct but clinically similar entity known as atypical adenomatous hyperplasia or atypical prostatic hyperplasia may be related to prostate cancer (Garnett and Oyasu 1989; Helpap 1980), it would be necessary to rule out this diagnosis in any epidemiologic study of BPH as a potential risk factor for prostate cancer. This is one of several reasons why lack of histologic confirmation of BPH is a serious weakness in an epidemiologic study examining BPH as a risk factor for prostate cancer. The study which found no increased risk compared prostate cancer incidence among men who had undergone transurethral prostatectomies (TURPs) for BPH with that in age-matched controls. The author justified his use of BPH patients who had undergone TURPs by noting that prostate cancer typically involves a part of the prostate not removed by TURP (McNeal 1969). However, the exclusion from the BPH cases of men with latent prostate cancer found at TURP may have created a bias in this study, since no similar exclusion of latent cancer could be made for the controls (Nomura and Kolonel 1992). Based on all evidence from both studies, it does not appear that BPH predisposes to prostate cancer.

Community-Based Urologic Studies

Two community-based studies of male urologic conditions have recently been started, one in Rochester, Minnesota and the other in Stirling, Scotland. Initial findings from the Stirling study have recently been published (Garraway et al. 1991). The two studies have similar protocols. Each is intended to describe the long-term course of urologic conditions among a randomly chosen sample of more than 2000 men, age 40 through 79 upon entry, who have not had prostate surgery, prostate cancer, or certain medical conditions (e.g., neurogenic bladder) that could interfere with urologic evaluation.

In each study, all men receive a questionnaire covering urologic symptoms, urologic interference with daily activities, psychological well-being, sexual functioning, health-care seeking behavior, and health-related worries and concerns. In addition, demographic, smoking, dietary, and beverage information is obtained. Urinary flow rate measurements are obtained on all men in each study.

In the Rochester study a randomly chosen subsample of 500 men was selected to undergo urologic evaluations including prostate size measurements by transrectal ultrasound, repeat urinary flow rate measurements, and several laboratory tests including prostate-specific antigen, and serum urea nitrogen. In the Stirling study the in-clinic evaluation was initially limited to men meeting certain criteria for symptoms or urinary flow rate (Garraway et al. 1991). Follow-up examinations on the men in these studies are planned.

The baseline phase of these studies will provide age-specific norms for symptoms, urinary flow rates, and prostate size by transrectal ultrasound. In addition it should be possible to determine relationships between prostate size, flow rate, symptoms, health-care-seeking behavior, and quality-of-life. Follow-up examinations should help delineate relationships between baseline information and measures of outcome such as BPH progression, surgical treatment, and complications of untreated disease.

This information should help provide a firmer base for counseling patients about what ranges of conditions are likely for them with and without treatment. It should be possible to project likely ranges of BPH evolution not only in terms of measurements such as flow rates, but also in terms of factors such as symptoms and extent to which symptoms interfere with daily activities. The latter is related to the concept of patient symptom preference, which Barry found to be critically important in making BPH treatment recommendations (Barry et al. 1988).

In summary, information on the development and progression of BPH in the absence of treatment is needed to guide treatment decisions. Community-based urologic studies can help provide this information. While baseline data will provide a substantial immediate addition to the literature, the true value of such studies will come from the long-term data which will emerge over time.

References

Abrams PH, Roylance J, Feneley RC (1976) Excretion urography in the investigation of prostatism. Br J Urol 48:681–684

Andersen JT, Vejlsgaard R (1980) The risk of inducing bacteriuria in urodynamic and uroradiological studies of men with prostatism. Scand J Urol Nephrol 14:229–232

Anderson JB, Grant JB F (1991) Postoperative retention of urine: a prospective urodynamic study. Br Med J 302:894–896

Armenian HK, Lilienfeld AM, Diamond EL, Bross ID (1974) Relation between benign prostatic hyperplasia and cancer of the prostate. A prospective and retrospective study. Lancet ii:115–117

Arrighi HM, Guess HA, Metter EJ, Fozard JL (1990) Symptoms and signs of prostatism as risk factors for prostatectomy. Prostate 16:253–261

Ball AJ, Feneley RC, Abrams PH (1981) The natural history of untreated "prostatism". Br J Urol 53:613–616

Barry MJ (1990a) Medical outcomes research and benign prostatic hyperplasia. Prostate [Suppl] 3:61–74

Barry MJ (1990b) Epidemiology and natural history of benign prostatic hyperplasia. Urol Clin North Am 17:495–507

Barry MJ, Mulley AG Jr, Fowler FJ, Wennberg JW (1988) Watchful waiting vs immediate transurethral resection for symptomatic prostatism. The importance of patients' preferences. JAMA 259:3010–3017

Bennett HS, Baggenstoss AH, Butt HR (1950) The testis, breast, and prostate of men who die of cirrhosis of the liver. Am J Clin Path 20:814–828

Berry SJ, Coffey DS, Walsh PC, Ewing LL (1984) The development of human benign prostatic hyperplasia with age. J Urol 132:474–479

Birkhoff JD (1983) Natural history of benign prostatic hypertrophy. In: Hinman F Jr (ed) Benign prostatic hypertrophy. Springer, Berlin Heidelberg New York, pp. 5–9

Birkhoff JD, Wiederhorn AR, Hamilton ML, Zinsser HH (1976) Natural history of benign prostatic hypertrophy and acute urinary retention. Urology 7:48–52

Clarke R (1937) The prostate and the endocrines - a control series. Br J Urol 9:254–271

Craigen AA, Hickling JD, Saunders CR, Carpenter RG (1969) Natural history of prostatic obstruction. A prospective survey. J R Coll Gen Pract 18:226–232

D'Aunoy R, Schenken JR, Burns EL (1939) The relative incidence of hyperplasia of the prostate in the white and colored races in Louisiana. South Med J 32:47–52

Drach GW, Layton TN, Binard WJ (1979) Male peak urinary flow rate: relationships to volume voided and age. J Urol 122:210–214

Franks LM (1974) Letter: Benign prostatic hyperplasia. Lancet ii:293

Frea B, Annoscia S, Stanta G, Lozzi C, Carmignani G (1987) Correlation between liver cirrhosis and benign prostatic hyperplasia: a morphological study. Urol Res 15:311–314

Garnett JE, Oyasu R (1989) Urologic evaluation of atypical prostatic hyperplasia. Urology 34 [6, Suppl]:66–69

Garraway WM, Collins GN, Lee RJ (1991) High prevalence of benign prostatic hypertrophy in the community. Lancet 338:469–471

Glynn RJ, Campion EW, Bouchard GR, Silbert JE (1985) The development of benign prostatic hyperplasia among volunteers in the Normative Aging Study. Am J Epidemiol 121:78–90

Gordon GG, Altman K, Southern AL, Rubin E, Lieber CS (1976) Effect of alcohol (ethanol) administration on sex hormone metabolism in normal men. N Engl J Med 295:793–797

Graversen PH, Gasser TC, Wasson JH, Hinman F Jr, Bruskewitz RC (1989) Controversies about indications for transurethral resection of the prostate. J Urol 141:475–481

Greenwald P, Kirmss V, Polan AK, Dick VS (1974) Cancer of the prostate among men with benign prostatic hyperplasia. J Natl Cancer Inst 53:335–340

Grosse H (1990) [Frequency, localization and associated disorders in urinary calculi. Analysis of 1671 autopsies in urolithiasis]. Z Urol Nephrol 83:469–474

Guess HA, Arrighi HM, Metter EJ, Fozard JL (1990) Cumulative prevalence of prostatism matches the autopsy prevalence of benign prostatic hyperplasia. Prostate 17:241–246

Hasner E (1962) Prostatic urinary infection. Acta Chir Scand [Suppl] 285:7–40

Helpap B (1980) The biological significance of atypical hyperplasia of the prostate. Virchows-Arch [Pathol Anat] 387:307–317

Hricak H, Jeffrey RB, Dooms GC, Tanagho EA (1987) Evaluation of prostate size: a comparison of ultrasound and magnetic resonance imaging. Urol Radiol 9:1–8

Jensen KM, Bruskewitz RC, Iversen P, Madsen PO (1983) Significance of prostatic weight in prostatism. Urol Int 38:173–178

Kaufman J, Dhakal M, Patel B, Hamburger R (1991) Community acquired acute renal failure. Am J Kidney Dis 17:191–198

Lytton B (1983) Interracial incidence of benign prostatic hypertrophy. In: Hinman F Jr (ed). Benign prostatic hypertrophy. Springer, Berlin Heidelberg New York, pp 22–26

McNeal JE (1969) Origin and development of carcinoma in the prostate. Cancer 23:24–34

McNeal JE (1978) Origin and evolution of benign prostatic enlargement. Invest Urol 15:340–345

McNeal JE (1990) Pathology of benign prostatic hyperplasia insight into etiology. Urol Clin North Am 17:477–486

Meyhoff HH, Hald T (1978) Are doctors able to assess prostatic size? Scand J Urol Nephrol 12:219–221

Meyhoff HH, Ingemann L, Nordling J, Hald T (1981) Accuracy in preoperative estimation of prostatic size. A comparative evaluation of rectal palpation, intravenous pyelography, urethral closure pressure profile recording and cystourethroscopy. Scand J Urol Nephrol 15:45–51

Nomura A, Kolonel LN (1992) Prostate cancer: a current perspective. Epidemiol Rev 14: (to be published)

Ohnishi K, Watanabe H, Ohe H (1987) Development of benign prostatic hypertrophy estimated from ultrasonic measurements with long-term follow-up. Tohoku J Exp Med 151:51–56

Powell PH, Smith PJ, Feneley RC (1980) The identification of patients at risk from acute retention. Br J Urol 52:520–522

Randall A (1931) Surgical pathology of prostatic obstruction. Williams and Willkins, Baltimore, pp 11–16

Robson MC (1966) Cirrhosis and prostatic neoplasms. Geriatrics 21:150–154

Sacks SH, Aparicio SA, Bevan A, Oliver DO, Will EJ, Davison AM (1989) Late renal failure due to prostatic outflow obstruction: a preventable disease. Br Med J 298:156–159

Sidney S, Quesenberry CP, Sadler MC, Guess HA, Lydick EG, Cattolica EV (1991a) Incidence of surgically treated benign prostatic hypertrophy and of prostate cancer among blacks and whites in a prepaid health care plan. Am J Epidemiol 134:825–829

Sidney S, Quesenberry C., Sadler MC, Lydick EG, Guess HA, Cattolica EV (1991b) Risk factors for surgically treated benign prostatic hyperplasia in a prepaid health care plan. Urology 38 [Suppl 1]:13–19

Spiro LH, Labay G, Orkin LA (1974) Prostatic infarction. Role in acute urinary retention. Urology 3:345–347

Stumpf HH, Wilens SL (1953) Inhibitory effects of portal cirrhosis of liver on prostatic enlargement. Arch Intern Med 91:304–309

Tolley DA, English PJ, Grigor KM (1987) Massive benign prostatic hyperplasia. J R Soc Med 80:777–778

Walsh PC (1986) Benign prostatic hyperplasia In: Walsh PC, Gittes RF, Perlmutter AD, Stamey TA (eds) Campbell's urology, 5th edn. Saunders, Philadelphia, pp 1248–1265

Walsh PC (1992) Benign prostatic hyperplasia. In: Walsh PC, Gittes RF, Perlmutter AD, Stamey TA (eds) Campbell's urology, 6th edn. Saunders, Philadelphia (to be published)

Watanabe H, Saitoh M, Mishina T, Igari D, Tanahashi Y, Harada K et al. (1977) Mass screening
    program for prostatic diseases with transrectal ultrasonotomography. J Urol 117:746–748
Williams RD, Blackard CE (1974) Benign prostatic hyperplasia and cancer of the prostate. Lancet
    ii:1265 (letter)

Pathogenesis of Benign Prostatic Hyperplasia

J.T.Grayhack, C.Lee and J.M.Kozlowski

Introduction

Benign prostatic hyperplasia (BPH) occurs in the great majority of adult human males with a prostate and testes who live long enough. The prevalence noted varies depending on the criteria employed for diagnosis; it is higher in most autopsy series employing histologic criteria than in clinical series employing gross anatomic assessments. Berry and associates (1984) summarized the evidence regarding the prevalence of BPH from interpretable reported autopsy studies available at the time. Although BPH was recognized infrequently in individuals in their 30s (8%), the prevalence increased rapidly from the fourth decade on. BPH is identifiable in over 40% of the men age 50–60 and 70% of men between 61 and 70 years of age. Gross enlargement of the prostate is recognized less frequently. Watanabe and associates (1984) identified prostatic enlargement, interpreted as BPH, on transrectal ultrasound evaluation in 37% of 1071 Japanese males over the age of 55. Glynn and associates (1985) observed that 78% of 2049 healthy men in a longitudinal Veterans Administration study had a diagnosis of BPH on symptomatic or physical evaluation by the age of 80. The discordance in autopsy and clinical data probably reflects the fact that gross enlargement of the prostate is identifiable in only about half the men with histologic evidence of hyperplasia (Isaacs 1990). In the consolidated autopsy data (Berry et al. 1984) the mean weight of the prostate only increased from 18 g to 31 g from the second to the eighth decade. Only a limited proportion of assessable glands with histologic evidence of BPH in men less than age 70 equaled or exceeded a 50% increase in the mean 18 g gland weight of a young adult (Grayhack 1992). The restricted magnitude of the weight gain should not be equated with lack of clinical significance, however, since a direct correlation between prostatic mass and clinical phenomena does not exist (Moore 1943). Clearly, BPH is progressively more prevalent as the human male with testes ages. The prevalence of the disease indicates a high probability that BPH is a pathophysiologic phenomenon. This probability is reinforced by the reproducibility of autopsy observations based on histologic criteria in populations with very different racial and environmental backgrounds (Fig. 1, Isaacs and Coffey 1989). In evaluating possible etiologic factors in the development of BPH the following deserve emphasis; (1) the previously identified concept of a pathophysiologic change; (2) the anatomic and pathologic characteristics of

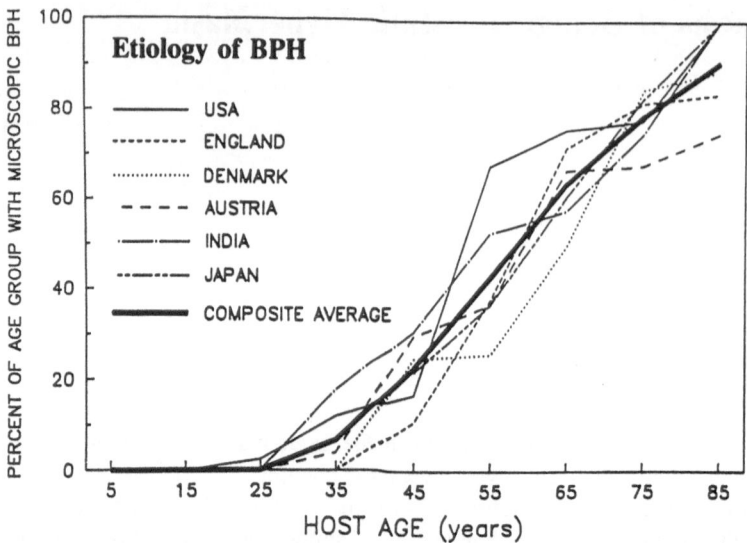

Fig. 1. Age-specific prevalence of BPH in various geographic male populations. (From Isaacs and Coffey 1989)

BPH as compared to normal prostatic growth; and (3) the probable relationship of normal physiologic phenomena controlling prostatic growth to the development of BPH.

Pathology

The important aspects of the pathologic changes that characterize BPH from the standpoint of pathogenesis, in addition to its almost certain development with progressive aging, are the following: (a) BPH is a regional disease; (b) in man the gross configuration of BPH is characterized by nodularity; and (3) the histologic composition of BPH is variegated within and between specimens. Hypotheses with regard to etiologic factors in BPH should take these observations into consideration.

Regional Development of BPH

The fact that BPH develops in the sub- and periurethral tissue has been recognized for more than half a century (see Hinman 1947). Various anatomic configurations have been proposed to describe the area that contains the tissues that undergo hyperplasia to produce BPH. According to McNeal (1990) the predominant site for the development of BPH is located not only periurethrally but also in the portion of the prostate adjacent to the proximal portion of the verumontanum and consequently the ejaculatory duct orifices. He has designated this the "transition zone." The other major site is the somewhat more proximal suburethral area. Recognizable BPH is a very uncommon phenomenon in the other regions of the prostate. Regional development of BPH suggests that tissues in these regions have either a different embryologic or programmed development or they are exposed to different environmental stimuli than other portions of the prostate. Both these considerations could be factors in the observed regional development of BPH.

Nodularity

BPH in man is characterized by localized foci of tissue growth that are frequently organized into distinct nodules. Early lesions with a nodular configuration have been identified in the periurethral area by several observers. As these lesions enlarge they compress the outer or peripheral, presumably normal, prostate and the so-called surgical capsule is formed. Recent observations (Lissner and Tisell 1979), confirmed by our own unreported experience, indicate that the peripheral prostate also increases in mass to some degree with age. Again the nodular development would seem to represent either regional intrinsic developmental differences in tissue or exposure to localized extrinsic factors or both.

Variegated Histologic Composition

Current observations indicate that cells constituting the stroma predominate in BPH (Bartsch et al. 1979; Shapiro et al. 1992). However, all elements of the normal prostate except elastic tissue may be variably involved in the nodular hyperplasia. Franks (1976) states that acinar and ductal epithelium and muscular and fibrous stroma can produce nodules of varying histologic composition which he characterizes as one of five types: (1) stromal (fibrous or fibrovascular); (2) fibromuscular; (3) muscular; (4) fibroadenomatous; and (5) fibromyoadenomatous. Nodules of different histologic types often coexist in the same prostate. Again the existence of localized hyperplasia that is histologically variegated in a given gland suggests exposure to localized extrinsic stimuli or intrinsic programmed development of the tissue involved.

Natural History

On the basis of age-related anatomic observations McNeal (1990) suggests two phases to the development of BPH in man. The initial phase, which is recognizable in some autopsy specimens obtained from men in their 30s, is the development of multiple small nodules or tissue foci; these seem to increase in number with limited progression in size for many years. Based on autopsy studies, McNeal

(1990) suggests that a second phase, characterized by a rapid expansive growth of some of these previously developed nodules, takes place. Clinical impressions and observations of control populations in drug studies also support a variable natural history including progression, stability, and probable regression for BPH and its physiologic effects (Glynn et al. 1985; Grayhack 1992; Isaacs 1990). All told, these scientifically challengeable observations support the suggestion that BPH may undergo a phasic growth which is similar chronologically but not necessarily genetically or physiologically to the initiation and promotion phenomena associated with the development of malignancy.

Physiological Considerations

Androgens

The prostate is a male accessory sex organ that is normally dependent on intact testicular function and androgen secretion and end organ metabolism for its development and growth. In selected animals the relationship between androgenic stimulation and the growth and function of the prostate is sufficiently predictable to permit this interrelationship to be employed as an androgen assay procedure (Mann and Lutwak-Mann 1981). In the human, the prostate undergoes increase in size at birth, puberty, and old age. The increase in mass that occurs at birth and puberty is related time-wise to physiologically induced stimulation of secretion of androgen by the testes. Endocrine evaluation of the aging male has disclosed no recognizable surge in androgen secretion to explain the observed prostatic growth. The available evidence indicates that serum levels of testosterone, in particular free testosterone, decrease with advancing age (Vermuelen et al. 1972). These observations are reinforced by urinary assays (Dorfman and Shipley 1956) and biologic studies. Taken together we conclude that, although androgen plays an important role in prostatic growth and function, androgen alone cannot be solely responsible for the commonly observed prostatic growth in old age. Indeed, it would appear that androgens constitute very proximate signals in a cascade of signaling events which culminate in the expression of various growth factors and/or their receptors (Traish and Wotiz 1987). Factors other than androgen must be important etiologically for the development and/or growth of BPH.

Systemic Proteins

Studies of sex hormone binding globulin (SHBG) and prolactin have provided evidence for their potential roles in prostatic growth. The evidence of a synergistic effect of prolactin on androgen-induced prostatic growth in rodents is extensive but a physiologically important role for this protein hormone in prostatic growth has not been established in animals and man (Lee and Grayhack 1989). The possible role of SHBG in prostatic growth has been suggested by two lines of evidence. First,

Rosner (1991) has found receptor sites for SHBG on human prostatic epithelial cells. The activated SHBG is able to induce cyclic AMP production in these cells. Second, BPH develops at a time when circulating free testosterone is declining but serum levels of SHBG are rising. The effect of SHBG, if any, will be a systemic one. However, the counterpart of SHBG in the seminal plasma is androgen-binding protein (ABP) which is derived from the Sertoli cells. A single gene is responsible for the synthesis of both the SHBG and the testicular ABP. Although SHBG and ABP have different glycosylation patterns, they cross react in radioimmunoassays (Cheng et al. 1984). Consequently the potential for both local and systemic prostatic stimulation exists.

The observations with regard to SHBG and prostatic epithelial cell interaction provide a potential generic pattern for the mechanism of signal transmission by a protein derived from an extrinsic source.

Growth Factors

Numerous growth factors including basic fibroblast growth factor (bFGF), transforming growth factor-α (TGF α), epidermal growth factor (EGF), keratinocyte growth factor (KGF), and a nerve growth factor-like protein (NGF) have been identified in prostatic tissue and cultures of normal and abnormal prostatic cells (Hofer et al. 1991; Sherwood et al. 1992; Peehl and Stamey 1991; Graham et al. 1992). KGF and NGF have been shown to be synthesized and secreted by stromal elements and to bind preferentially to high-affinity receptors located on adjacent epithelial cells (Rubin et al. 1989; Bottaro et al. 1990; Graham et al. 1992). The distribution of these and other growth factors/receptors provide potential mechanisms for autocrine and paracrine cellular interaction that are being studied extensively. Moreover, the heparan sulfate proteoglycans which are abundant in the prostatic extracellular matrix may avidly sequester heparin-binding growth factors, such as bFGF, protect such moieties from proteolytic degradation/inactivation, and facilitate their slow sustained impact on sensitive target cells (Sherwood et al. 1992). The role of intrinsic prostatic growth factors, singly or in combination, in the development and growth of BPH is likely to be, like androgen, essential but not critical. Overall the tissue studies that have attempted to identify growth mechanisms and products in BPH have supported the concept that BPH results from alterations in regulation of normal prostatic growth mechanisms.

Tissue Analysis

Despite the reduction in circulating testosterone levels in the aging male, the tissue levels of dihydrotestosterone (DHT) in the prostatic adenoma and the peripheral prostate are in a range that approximates or exceeds that of young males and are comparable (Walsh et al. 1983). These DHT tissue concentrations and the associated prostatic growth with decreasing free serum testosterone levels are paradoxical. The persistent role of androgen in the maintenance of at least epithelial cell growth and function (e.g. prostate-specific antigen, PSA) in BPH seems clearly established by histologic evidence derived from autopsy observations of endocrine manipulated patients and clinical studies employing suppression of testicular function (Wendel et al. 1972; Peters and Walsh 1987). Although an excessive homogeneous, not nodular, hyperplastic growth of the prostate can be produced in the dog by administration of supraphysiologic amounts of androgen (Garnett et al. 1992), evidence of an initiating, or even independent promoting role of androgen has not been presented in humans.

Efforts to identify unique chemical and biochemical characteristics of BPH have not yielded insightful information (Grayhack and Kozlowski 1991). Many of these investigative endeavors, including steroid content and receptor studies, have employed the peripheral prostate as "normal" or controlled tissue. Since the peripheral prostate is almost certainly exposed to systemic accessory sex gland factors influencing growth phenomena and may have different responses to them, observations resulting from these efforts must be interpreted with caution. No difference in the concentration of enzymes involved in steroid metabolism including 5α-reductase, 3α-hydroxyoxidoreductase, 4β-hydroxysteroid oxidoreductase, and 17β-hydroxysteroid oxidoreductase have been identified consistently between BPH and peripheral prostate in the often conflicting reports in the literature. Phosphatase activity has been found to be increased in BPH tissue (Brendler et al. 1985), whereas other cytoplasmic enzymes, including lactic dehydrogenase and alkaline phosphatase, have not.

Accessory Sex Gland Age-Related Organ Weight and Secretory Status

In animals, weight and histology of selected accessory glands have been employed to assay systemic factors, primarily the endocrine status, as they relate to accessory sex gland growth and function (Mann and Lutwak-Mann 1981). Quantitative assay of selected secretory products, for example, fructose and citric acid, provides an opportunity to obtain additional insights into the effects of systemic factors controlling or altering accessory sex gland growth. In selected animals, the level of fructose in the accessory sex gland secretion correlates directly with systemic androgen levels. Secretion of citric acid in the prostate of rodents depends on androgen stimulation but is modifiable by other endocrine secretions such as prolactin and indirectly by estrogens. The combination of assessment of selected endocrine-dependent secretory activities and gravimetric indicators of accessory sex gland growth in the human male with increasing age indicates the following: (1) the weight of the seminal vesical, an accessory sex gland only rarely the site of significant pathology, is maintained at about a stable level from postpuberty to old age; the fructose concentration in the seminal vesical fluid, by contrast, decreases progressively with age from a very high to a low concentration; (Grayhack 1961) and (2) the citric acid concentration in the digitally expressed prostatic fluid of 40–60 year old males is higher than the concentration in both younger and older age groups. The citric acid concentration of a group of men 20–40 as compared to those over 60 is not significantly different. Contrastingly, acid phosphatase and lactate dehydrogenase concentrations in human prostatic fluid show a progressive decline with age (Grayhack and Kropp 1965). The maintenance of weight of the seminal vesical and the increased or maintained secretion of citric acid by the prostate provide evidence of accessory sex gland stimulation as the human male ages. The progressive age-related decrease in fructose in seminal vesical fluid and acid phosphatase concentration in prostatic fluid provides strong support for the probability that direct androgen stimulation is unlikely to be the critical factor in progressive prostatic growth with age. Since multiple human accessory organs are involved in these observations, the likelihood of a systemic accessory sex gland stimulating factor(s) that is not androgen seems substantial. However, an additional, and perhaps very important, role for possible local exposure to these stimulating factors and an essential role for androgen in their end organ effects certainly deserves continuing serious consideration.

Etiologic Considerations

The etiologic factors that result in BPH in man have been the subject of intense evaluation and speculation. A wide variety of etiologic considerations have been proposed. These have included hypotheses that center on neoplastic, inflammatory, circulatory, metabolic and nutritional factors and hormonal alterations (Mostofi and Thompson 1963). In recent years (Isaacs and Coffey 1989), the efforts to understand the pathogenesis of BPH have centered essentially in two areas; (1) studies to identify changes in steroid hormone secretion and metabolism and (2) efforts to identify and understand the normal and perhaps abnormal mechanisms of stromal epithelial interaction. Isaacs and Coffey have recently proposed the "stem cell hypothesis" in which cell proliferation and cell death rates are important concepts. Overall the conviction that alteration in and/or abnormal stimulation of normal prostatic growth mechanisms are essential to the development of BPH is basic to these etiologic proposals.

The concept of a primary role for stromal alterations in integrating and possibly promoting BPH has been proposed and supported intermittently for well over half a century (Reischauer 1925). In glands that are judged pathologically to be in the early phase of BPH development, nodules located primarily in the sub- and periurethral areas are a common easily recognizable abnormality. Transition zone nodules are also observed frequently but are less discrete (McNeal 1990). The majority of the periurethral nodules are stromal or have minimal glandular content (McNeal 1990). These observations coupled with the recognition that stromal cells usually predominate in BPH, as compared to epithelial cells, have served to increase the perception that the initiating and perhaps promoting events that lead to the development and progression of BPH may be centered in induced or spontaneous stromal changes. The probable primary role for stroma in prostate development and possibly growth is supported by Cunha's (Cunha et al. 1980) demonstration that normal mouse urogenital sinus mesenchyme stimulates bladder epithelial cells obtained from androgen-insensitive mice that lack androgen receptor to develop prostate-like glandular epithelium. As indicated previously, identification of a variety of cellular proteins in prostatic tissue and secretions and in the culture media of normal and abnormal cells provides potential autocrine and paracrine mechanisms for integrated stromal-epithelial interaction and directed cellular response. Prostatic stroma has been identified as a source of a heparin-binding growth factor, probably identical to bFGF (Story et al. 1989; Jacobs et al. 1988). In vivo observations in mice transfected with *int*-2 gene, encoding a 27 kD a protein homologous with bFGF, demonstrated a marked increase in prostate volume compared to normal animals. The prostatic response to androgen ablation and administration of these mice indicated the persistent essential role of androgen in the growth of their accessory sex glands (Tutrone et al. 1991). Local exposure of the ventral prostate of Sprague-Dawley rats to bFGF-matrigel complex results in unilateral increased prostatic weight. In vitro observations in the rat indicate that bFGF is a direct mitogen for stroma (Marengo et al. 1992) but not for epithelial cells. TGF-α is produced by and stimulates proliferation of androgen-independent human prostatic cancer cell lines in vitro (Hofer et al. 1991). Impressive in vivo evidence of an effect of EGF on prostate growth has been recently presented in mice subjected to sialoadenectomy (Liu et al. 1992). Resulting reduction in prostatic weight was restored by administration of exogenous EGF. High and low affinity EGF binding was demonstrable in the prostate. Additionally EGF is an important component of the media used to achieve prostatic epithelial cell growth in vitro (McKeehan et al. 1984). Conditioned media of human stromal cells will stimulate BPH epithelial cell growth in vitro (Sherwood et al. 1992). These examples of this expanding body of information with regard to potential mechanisms of interaction between the various cellular components of the prostate are cited to reinforce the probability that, at one phase or another of abnormal growth, these interactions could be important or critical components. However the probability that these factors alone represent a critical event in the initiating phase of BPH seems small.

    The etiologic considerations that have received the most intense effort and scrutiny over the years with regard to the development and progression of BPH have focused on the possible effects of primary or interactive hormonal changes on the prostate. Pursuit of a possible endocrine etiology of BPH has clearly been reinforced by the critical role of endocrine secretions, primarily testicular, in the development and growth of the normal prostate and the critical role of functioning testes in the development of BPH. As previously cited, demonstration of normal or possibly slightly increased levels of DHT in BPH tissue served to fuel pursuit of possible endocrine factors in its initiation and progression. The observations indicating that a homogeneous, diffuse and, just recently, cystic BPH could be induced in the dog by administration of androgens alone or combined with estrogens, served to reinforce this concept (Garnett et al. 1992; Juniewicz et al. 1992). Consequently changes in absolute or relative levels of primary steroid hormones that correlated with the presence of clinically significant BPH have been sought with repetitious persistence, employing new information and technologies as they have become available. Identifying age-matched controls for these efforts has been a major problem because of the prevalence of BPH in the elderly. As indicated earlier serum testosterone levels fall with aging. However in some studies, not all, this fall is not significant until 70 years of age or older. Serum DHT levels also have been observed to decline with age. By contrast, high-affinity SHBG increases with aging; physiologically active free testosterone is consequently demonstrably and disproportionately decreased. These observations, coupled with a stable or slightly increased serum estrogen (estrone; estradiol) level in aging males, results in an increased estrogen androgen ratio in this group of men (Neubauer 1983; Karr and Murphy 1983). The literature in these cited summaries and the recent assessment by Partin et al. (1991) of the relationship between serum hormone levels and the volume of BPH in patients subjected to radical prostatectomy failed to identify persistent, acceptably documented, important steroid hormone changes that differentiate the aged human male with BPH from his comparably aged counterpart in whom BPH is not documented to be present. Partin et al. (1991) demonstrated an age associated decrease in serum free testosterone, androstenedione, 5-androstenediol, 17-hydroxypregnenolone, and dehydroepiandrosterone (DHEA) and its sulphate (DHEAS). Increases were noted in serum SHBG, luteinizing hormonal (LH), and follicle stimulating hormone (FSH) levels. When corrected for age the BPH volume in the surgically removed specimens correlated positively with serum free testosterone, estradiol, and estriol but not with the DHT levels. The findings of this study were interpreted to suggest that androgen, acting synergistically with estrogen, may be a factor responsible for persistent stimulation of BPH. Isaacs and Coffey (1989) summarized the probable role of DHT, and also testosterone, in the pathogenesis of BPH by indicating that androgen is a necessary but not sufficient condition for its development (see also Grayhack 1976).

The rather extensive data with regard to systemic levels of androgenic steroids in elderly males and the tissue levels of DHT in both the portion of the prostate that represents compressed "normal" prostate and BPH constitutes a paradox. The unequivocal evidence of tissue stimulation in the abnormal periurethral prostatic tissue and the less well established but probable stimulation of the tissue of the so-called surgical capsule supports the probability that this accumulated DHT is physiologically active. The "necessary" role of androgen and the testis in the promotion of growth of the prostate of the aging male adds evidence to support the hypothesis that the initiating and critical event in the development of BPH produces the local changes in the prostate that lead to the paradoxical physiologically important accumulation of intracellular DHT and perhaps synergize its effect. The limited but definite decrease in stimulation and size of BPH epithelial cells associated with decreases in systemic androgen levels (Wendel et al. 1972; Peters and Walsh 1987) adds evidence supporting the physiologic significance of the intracellular androgen concentrations observed. The previously cited observations of biological indicators of accessory sex gland stimulation in men considered in relation to age-associated prostatic growth stimulation (BPH) supports the probability of systemic and/or local physiologic mechanisms to produce synergized androgen-mediated prostatic growth (Fig. 2).

As observations supporting the paradox of increased androgen-mediated prostatic stimulation in the presence of diminished systemic androgen have accumulated, the possibility of a critical role for a systemic and/or regional protein stimulating prostatic growth has begun to receive increasing consideration. Evidence has been accumulating supporting the suggestion that the testis has the capability of secreting a substance(s) that will synergize androgen-mediated accessory sex gland growth. Radiation of the testis of elderly dogs with BPH reduced the size of their BPH compared to observations in non-radiated controlled dogs (Grayhack 1985). Serum levels of testosterone and estradiol were similar in dogs with radiated as compared to nonradiated testes, suggesting the role of a nonandrogenic testicular factor in this phenomenon. Administration of supraphysiologic amounts of DHT and testosterone to rats with testes has produced increased prostatic growth as compared to rats castrated at the time androgen administration was initiated (Dalton et al. 1990; Darras et al. 1992). The serum levels of LH and, in DHT-treated rats, of testosterone indicate essentially complete suppression of normal Leydig cell androgenic steroid secretion in testis bearing rats. Excessive prostatic growth has been observed in adult rats subjected to propylthiouracil-induced hypothyroidism transiently during the neonatal period. A marked proliferation of the testicular tubules results in increased testis size and weight in these animals. The serum testosterone levels, however, are comparable to normal rats (Cooke and Meisami 1991). Juniewicz et al. (1992) recently reported a significantly greater prostatic growth and incidence of BPH in 5 year old beagles with testes as compared to dogs with documented physiologic replacement of

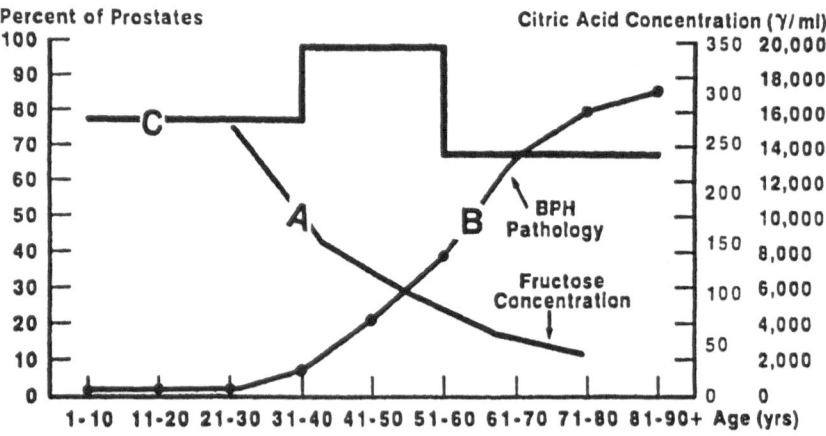

Fig. 2. Three biologic indicators of accessory sex gland stimulation in the human as related to age. *A* seminal vesicle fluid fructose concentration (from Grayhack 1961); *B* prevalence of BPH (from Berry et al. 1984), and *C* prostatic fluid citric acid concentration (from Grayhack and Kropp 1965)

androgen (testosterone) and estrogen (estradiol) after castration at 6 months of age. Additionally, in vitro experiments in our laboratory have repeatedly demonstrated protein fractions of the semen that stimulate proliferation of human BPH epithelial and stromal cells. One of these proteins, with a molecular weight of approximately 35 kDa was not present in the semen of vasectomized males. Overall the evidence to support the hypothesis that the testis produces a nonandrogenic factor that synergizes the growth promoting effect of androgen on the prostate is accumulating from a variety of experimental observations. This factor is very probably a protein involved in testicular tubular interactions and function. The hypothesized testicular protein prostate stimulating factor has two potential secretory pathways, systemic and regional (semen). Local exposure of the prostate to this testicular factor could play a critical role in the initiation and/or promotion of BPH. The proposed testicular nonandrogenic accessory sex gland stimulating factor offers a reasonable explanation for the regional (periurethral) and localized (nodular) growth and the variegated histology that characterizes human BPH. Additionally the cited observations with regard to SHBG binding to and interacting with prostatic epithelial cells (Rosner 1991) provides support for another potential source of a prostate stimulating protein. The rising serum levels of SHBG with aging in humans add to the interest in this protein. A relationship or interaction of systemic and testicular protein growth signals is a possibility that warrants the consideration it is receiving.

In summary, BPH occurs in almost all men with a prostate and functioning testes if they survive long enough. In vivo and in vitro observations of paracrine and autocrine growth mechanisms have provided evidence that prostatic growth is the result of a complex interaction of extrinsic and intrinsic cellular control mechanisms. The predominant extrinsic growth altering factors recognized as affecting the prostate have been steroid sex hormones. At this time the evidence seems to support a stable, necessary, but not critical role for these hormones in the growth processes associated with the development and progression of BPH. Evidence supporting the secretion of a nonsteroidal prostate stimulating substance by the testes is accumulating. This substance(s) provides another potential extrinsic agent that warrants consideration as the critical initiating and/or promoting stimulus for BPH. A possible role of SHBG as an extrinsic prostate stimulating growth factor also warrants continuing evaluation. Additionally, intrinsic alterations in growth mechanisms or cellular responses are receiving and warrant continued consideration as significant etiologic factors for BPH.

References

Bartsch G, Muller HR, Oberholzer M, Rohr HP (1979) Light microscopic stereological analysis of the normal human prostate and of benign prostatic hyperplasia. J Urol 122:487–491

Berry SJ, Coffey DS, Walsh PC, Ewing LL (1984) The development of human benign prostatic hyperplasia with age. J Urol 132:474–477

Bottaro D, Rubin J, Ron D, Finch P, Florio C, Aaronson S (1990) Characterization of the receptor for keratinocyte growth factor. J Biol Chem 265:12767–12770

Brendler CB, Follansbee AL, Isaacs JT (1985) Discrimination between normal, hyperplastic and malignant human prostatic tissue by enzymatic profiles. J Urol 133:495–501

Cheng CY, Frick J, Gunsalus GL, Musto NA, Bardin CW (1984) Human testicular androgen binding protein shares immunodeterminants with serum testosterone-estradiol binding globulin. Endocrinology 114:1395

Cooke PS, Meisami E (1991) Early hypothyroidism in rats causes increased adult testis and reproductive organ size but does not change testosterone levels. Endocrinology 129:237–243

Cunha GR, Lung B, Reese B (1980) Glandular epithelial induction by embryonic mesenchyme in adult bladder epithelium of BALB/C mice. Invest Urol 17:302

Dalton DP, Lee C, Huprikar S, Chmiel JS, Grayhack JT (1990) Non-androgenic role of testis in enhancing ventral prostate growth in rats. Prostate 16:225–233

Darras FS, Lee C, Huprikar S, Rademaker AW, Grayhack JT (1992) Evidence for a non-androgenic role of testis and epididymis in androgen-supported growth of the rat ventral prostate. J Urol 148: 432–440

Dorfman RI, Shipley RA (1956) Androgens. Wiley, New York, pp 397–399

Franks LM (1976) Benign prostatic hyperplasia: gross and microscopic anatomy. In: Grayhack JT, Wilson JD, Scherbenske MJ (eds) Benign prostatic hyperplasia: NIAMDD workshop proceedings, 20–21 Feb 1975. US Department of Health, Education, and Welfare publication no (NIH) 76–1113, pp 63–89

Garnett J, Lim D, Grayhack JT (1992) (to be published)

Glynn RJ, Campion EW, Bouchard GR, Silbert JE (1985) The development of benign prostatic hyperplasia among volunteers in the normative aging study. Am J Epidemiol 121:78–90

Graham CW, Lynch JH, Djakiew D (1992) Distribution of nerve growth factor-like protein and nerve growth factor receptor in human benign prostatic hyperplasia and prostatic adenocarcinoma. J Urol 147:1444–1447

Grayhack JT (1961) Changes with aging in human seminal vesicle fluid fructose concentration and seminal vesicle weight. J Urol 86:142–148

Grayhack JT (1972) Reflections on the etiology of benign prostatic hypertrophy. (Presented in Urological Research Papers in honor of William Wallace Scott). Plenum, New York, pp 39–50

Grayhack JT (1992) BPH: the scope of the problem. Cancer (in press)

Grayhack JT, Kozlowski J (1991) Benign prostatic hyperplasia. In: Grayhack JT, Howards SS, Duckett JW (eds) Gillenwater JY, Adult and pediatric urology, 2nd edn. Mosby Year Book, St Louis, pp 1211–1276

Grayhack JT, Kropp KA (1965) Changes with aging in prostatic fluid: Citric acid, acid phosphatase and lactic dehydrogenase concentration in man. J Urol 93:258–262

Hinman F (1947) The obstructive prostate. JAMA 135:136–141

Hofer DR, Sherwood ER, Bromberg WD, Mendelsohn J, Lee C, Kozlowski JM (1991) Autonomous growth of androgen-independent human prostatic carcinoma cells: role of transforming growth factor alpha. Cancer Res 54:2780–2785

Isaacs JT (1990) Importance of the natural history of benign prostatic hyperplasia in the evaluation of pharmacologic intervention. Prostate Suppl 3:1–7

Isaacs JT, Coffey DS (1989) Etiology and disease process of benign prostatic hyperplasia. Prostate Suppl 2:33–50

Jacobs SC, Story MT, Sasse J, Lawson RK (1988) Characterization of growth factors derived from the rat ventral prostate. J Urol 139:1106–1110

Juniewicz PE, Berry SJ, Coffey DS, Strandberg JD, Zirkin BR, Ewing LL (1992) The requirement of the testes in the development of benign prostatic hyperplasia (BPH) in the beagle. J Urol 147:249A

Karr JP, Murphy GP (1983) Cellular growth and hormone receptors. In: Hinman F Jr (ed) Benign prostatic hypertrophy. Springer, Berlin Heidelberg New York, pp 193–214

Lee C, Grayhack JT (1989) Prolactin and the prostate in animal models. In: Nagasawa H (ed) Prolactin and lesions in breast, uterus, and prostate. CRC Press, Boca Raton, pp 177–186

Lissner KH, Tisell LE (1979) The weight of the human prostate. Scand J Urol Nephrol 13:137–143

Liu AHY, Davis RJ, Flores C, Menon M, Seethalakshmi L (1992) Epidermal growth factor (EGF): receptor binding and effects on the sex accessory organs of sexually mature male mice. J Urol 147:214A

Mann T, Lutwak-Mann C (1981) Male reproductive function and semen. Springer, Berlin Heidelberg New York.

Marengo SR, Wang Xiao-Huai, Pistors LP, Chung LWK (1992) Regulation of growth of the normal prostate: effects of epidermal and basic fibroblast growth factors in vivo and in vitro. J Urol 147:248A

McKeehan WL, Adams PS, Rosser MP (1984) Direct mitogenic effects of insulin, epidermal growth factor, glucocorticoid, cholera toxin, unknown pituitary factors and possible prolactin, but not androgen, on normal rat prostate epithelial cells in serum-free, primary cell culture. Cancer Res 44:1998–2010

McNeal JE (1988) Normal histology of the prostate. Am J Surg Pathol 12:619–633

McNeal J (1990) Pathology of benign prostatic hyperplasia. Urol Clin North Am 17:477–486

Moore RA (1943) Benign hypertrophy of the prostate: a morphological study. J Urol 50:680–710

Mostofi FK, Thomson RV (1963) Benign hyperplasia of the prostate gland. In: Campbell M (ed) Urology, 2nd edn. Saunders, Philadelphia, pp 1101–1157, 1963

Neubauer BL (1983) Endocrine and cellular inductive factors in the development of human benign prostatic hypertrophy. In: Hinman F Jr (ed) Benign prostatic hypertrophy. Springer, Berlin Heidelberg New York, pp 179–192

Partin AW, Oesterling JE, Epstein JI, Horton R, Walsh PC (1991) Influence of age and endocrine factors on the volume of benign prostatic hyperplasia. J Urol 145:405–409

Peehl D, Stamey T (1991) Fibroblast growth factors can replace epidermal growth factor for a clonal proliferation of human prostatic epithelial cells. J Urol 145:331A

Peters CA, Walsh PC (1987) The effect of natarelin acetate, a luteinizing-hormone-releasing hormone agonist, on benign prostatic hyperplasia. N Engl J Med 317:599–604

Reischauer F (1925) Die Entstehung der sogenannten Prostatahypertrophie. Virchows Arch [Pathol Anat] 256:357–389

Rosner W (1991) Plasma steroid-binding proteins. Endocrinol Metab Clin North Am 20: 697–720

Rubin JS, Osada H, Finch PW, Taylor WG, Rudikoff S, Aaronson SA (1989) Purification and characterization of a newly identified growth factor specific for epithelial cells. PNAS 86:802–806

Shapiro E, Hartanto V, Lepor H (1992) Quantifying the smooth muscle content of the prostate using double-immunoenzymatic staining and color assisted image analysis. J Urol 147:1167–1170

Sherwood ER, Fong CJ, Lee C, Kozlowski JM (1992) Basic fibroblast growth factor: a potent mediator of stromal growth in the human prostate. Endocrinology 130:2955–2963

Story MT, Livingston B, Baeten L, Swartz SJ, Jacobs SC, Begun FP, Lawson RK (1989) Cultured human prostate-derived fibroblasts produce a factor that stimulates their growth with properties indistinguishable from basic fibroblast growth factor. Prostate 15:355–365

Story MT, Hopp KA, Lawson RK (1992) Growth of cultured prostatic stromal cells is regulated by basic fibroblast growth factor and transforming growth factor-ß1. J Urol 147:242A

Traish AM, Wotiz HH (1987) Prostatic epidermal growth factor receptors and their regulation by androgens. Endocrinology 121:1461–1467

Tutrone RF, Ball RA, Orvitz DM, Leder P, Ritchie JP (1991) Benign prostatic hyperplasia in a transgenic mouse: a hormonally responsive investigatory model. Surg Forum 42:697–699

Vermuelen A, Rubens R, Verdonch L (1972) Testosterone secretion and metabolism in male senescence. J Clin Endocrinol Metab 34: 730–735

Walsh PC, Hutchins GM, Ewing LL (1983) Tissue content of dihydro-testosterone in human prostatic hyperplasia is not supranormal. J Clin Invest 72:1772–1777

Watanabe, H, Ohe H, Inaba T, Itakura Y, Saitoh M, Nakao M (1984) A mobile mass screening unit for prostatic disease. Prostate 5: 559–565

Wendel E, Brannen GE, Putong PB, Grayhack JT (1972) The effect of orchietomy and estrogens on benign prostatic hyperplasia. J Urol 108:116–119

Benign Prostatic Hypertrophy: Standards and Guidelines

W.K.Mebust

Introduction

Patient care guidelines have always been available to the practicing physician. They come in the form of textbooks, professorial opinions, consensus of the experts, algorithms, and decision trees, etc. These guidelines have identified practices that are considered to be standard and acceptable which in turn, were determined by whatever practices were in common use at the particular time. Guidelines have been referred to as practice policies, standards of care, practice parameters, etc. The simplest method of guideline development, whether it involves individuals or groups, requires experts to process in their heads all the important information and requires anybody using this guideline to take the experts' opinion on faith.

The science of medicine has expanded tremendously in recent years. New complex diagnostic and therapeutic modalities have become available to the physician, who must take into consideration these new modalities and apply them to a specific situation while being aware of the good and bad outcomes that may occur. This can be an extremely complex task and there can be no pretention that the experts' have reasoned through the problem in an analytical fashion. Rather, the presumption is made that the experts can arrive at accurate answers intuitively. Therefore, the physicians dependence upon implicit guidelines does not necessarily mean that he will provide his patient appropriate care.

Medical specialities societies recently have become involved in developing practice policies which would include guidelines, standards, and strategies for patient management to assist the physician in clinical decision making. The number of physician organizations actively involved in developing practice policies has increased dramatically from one in 1937 to over 26 in 1989 (Kelly and Kellie 1990). Not only have these practice policies addressed appropriate indications for diagnostic and therapeutic modalities, but they have also been influenced by public policy discussions regarding quality, utilization, and cost of medical care.

Guidelines were developed for cardiac pacemaker implantation and had a tremendous effect upon the use of this procedure. Greenspan et al. (1988) reviewed retrospectively the appropriateness of indications for Medicare-reimbursed cardiac pacemaker implants performed at 30 hospitals in Philadelphia, during the first 6 months of 1983. Based on this study, a panel determined that 44% of the implants were definitely indicated, 35% possibly indicated and 20% not indicated. This resulted in a publication of a practice policy in 1984, developed by the

Joint Task Force of the American Heart Association and the American College of Cardiology (Guidelines 1964). The impact of this practice policy was a 27.9% reduction in the rate of permanent pacemaker implantation observed between 1983 and 1986.

In 1989, the Omnibus Budget Reconciliation Act passed by Congress included the provision for a new health care agency. This was the Agency for Health Care Policy and Research (AHCPR) which was placed in the Public Health Division of the Department of Health and Human Services. Congress mandated that the Department would undertake outcomes research but included a forum to develop practice policies or patient care guidelines. This stimulated many organizations to immediately begin developing practice policies for patient care. These organizations included local medical societies, third-party payers, physician review organizations, and a marked increased activity among the medical specialty societies.

It became apparent that there must be some consensus as to what were the proper attributes of a practice policy and what was the preferred method in developing such practice policies. AHCPR asked the Institute of Medicine (IOM) to develop such attributes (Field and Lohr 1990). The IOM concluded that:

1. The guidelines should have validity and that, if they were followed, this would lead to the expected health and cost outcomes projected for them.
2. The guidelines should have reliability and reproducibility and that, in a given situation, most physicians would do what was recommended by the guidelines; thus, they should also have clinical applicability and clinical flexibility.
3. The guidelines should be clearly written and a multi-disciplinary approach process should be included so that all groups affected would have participation in developing the guidelines.
4. The guidelines would have scheduled reviews to include new knowledge and revise the guidelines if unexpected consequences developed.
5. Finally, there should be accurate documentation as to the rationale in developing the policy.

The American Medical Association formed a partnership between itself and the major medical societies and also established a much larger forum for all those interested in developing patient care guidelines so that there would be an exchange of ideas and points of view in developing appropriate patient care policies.

In contrast to the implicit method most commonly used, Dr. David Eddy suggested that there be an explicit approach to patient care policies (Eddy 1990). The implicit approach accepts the beliefs of experts without requiring any description of the evidence considered, the consequences of different opinions, or the value judgments between the choice option. The explicit approach holds that such descriptions are essential to accurate assessment of a practice policy and the intelligent use of this policy.

The explicit approach is much more time-consuming, expensive, and complicated. It was adopted by the American Urological Association (AUA), in 1990, as they began to develop urologic care practice policies including the management of benign prostatic hypertrophy (BPH).

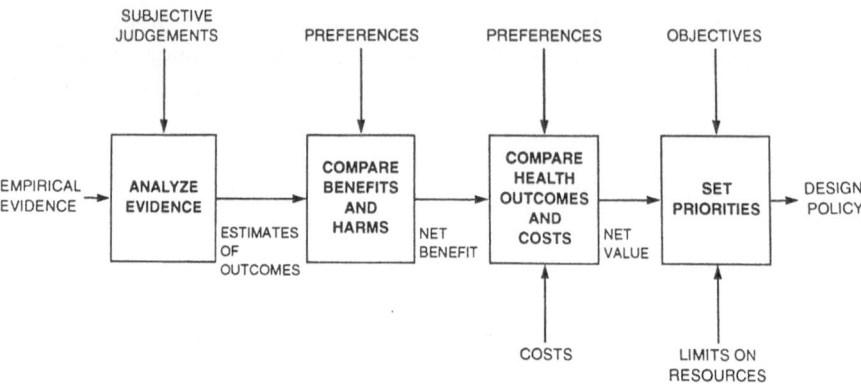

Fig. 1. The paradigm developed by Dr. David Eddy for the development of explicit guidelines (Eddy 1992)

The AUA committees were to develop guidelines which were to be laid open and the basis of the policy recommendations were to be documented. Formal methods could be applied to support any complicated steps in the design of the policy, such as analysis of the evidence or estimation of risks and benefits. This would allow any individual to carefully evaluate the policy and understand the rationale and scientific basis for the recommendation. A panel would look at the evidence, as it existed in the literature, and where evidence did not exist to help them in their recommendation, they would use expert opinion. However, it would be clearly stated in the document that expert opinion was used and who the experts were. The panel would then estimate the outcomes and compare the harms and benefits. At this point, they would also take into consideration the patient care preferences. The third step would be to compare the health care outcomes and the relative cost. If society had an unlimited amount of money to use for health care, this would not be an issue; but since health care now consumes 12% of our gross national product and is estimated to go up to 17% within the decade, it becomes quite apparent that cost must be considered. Taking both cost and the health outcomes into consideration, a set of priorities could be developed and a policy designed (Fig. 1). Setting priorities, however, would not necessarily be the charge of a panel developing a guideline, as it is really the consensus of society as to which priorities are important. Should monies be invested, for example, in the health care of children as opposed to the health care problems of the aging?

Once a health care policy or guideline has been developed, it needs to be evaluated as to its impact upon patients, physicians, and those bearing the costs of health care. An assessment would have to be undertaken to determine if the health care policy actually did effect practice patterns.

Table 1. Agency for Health Care Policy and Research's A BPH Panel

---

Urologists
  John McConnell, M.D., Chairman - Dallas, Texas
  Claus Roehrborn, M.D. Consultant - Dallas, Texas
  Peter Albertsen, M.D., Consultant-Farmington, Connecticut
  Winston K. Mebust, M.D., Consultant - Kansas City, Kansas
  Logan Holtgrewe, M.D., Consultant - Annapolis, Maryland
  Sherwood Denton, M.D. - Phoenix, Arizona
  Anton Bueschen, M.D. - Birmingham, Alabama
  John Lange, M.D. - Fort Smith, Arkansas
  Jerry Blaivas, M.D. - New York, New York
  Reginald Bruskewitz, M.D. - Madison, Wisconsin
  Stephen Sacks, M.D. - Los Angeles, California Internists
Internists
  Michael Barry, M.D., - Boston, Massachusetts
  John Wason, M.D., - White River Junction, Vermont Family Practice
Family Practice
  Richard Roberts, M.D. - Madison, Wisconsin Radiologist
Radiologist
  Bruce McClennan, M.D. - St. Louis, Missouri Nursing
Nursing
  Nancy Reilly, B.S., M.S., R.N. - Philadelphia, Pennsylvania

---

Guideline Panel

The Panel on the Diagnosis and Management of Benign Prostatic Hypertrophy, established by the AUA in 1990 with Dr. John McConnell as chairman, was taken over by the AHCPR and greatly expanded (Table 1). The BPH panel adopted many of Dr. Eddy's objectives which were laid out as eight specific tasks:

1. Formulating the assessment problem
2. Identifying it and documenting the available evidence
3. Synthesizing the evidence to estimate the magnitudes of the outcomes (harms and benefits)
4. Comparing harms and benefits
5. Estimating cost of an intervention
6. Comparing health outcomes and costs
7. Setting priorities
8. Designing a health policy

The available evidence is summarized in an 'evidence table' and the harms and benefits are summarized in a 'balance sheet' (Table 2).

Table 2. Assessment of Alternative Treatments. Balance sheet of harms and benefits for various therapeutic modalities used to treat benign prostatic hyperplasia (BPH). Preliminary data from Agency for Health Care Policy and Research (AHCPR) BPH Panel

	Watchful waiting	Transurethral surgery	Balloon dilation	α-Blocker
Benefits				
Chance of experiencing an improvement in your symptoms	31%–55%	75%–96%	37%–76%	59%–86%
Amount of symptom improvement you may experience[a]	+	++++	++	++
Risks and complications				
Chance of experiencing immediate complications as a result of the treatment[b]	None	6%–32% (includes complications during surgery, bleeding, infection, temporary inability to urinate)	2%–10% (includes complications during dilation, bleeding, infection, temporary inability to urinate)	3%–45% (includes dizziness, lightheadedness, low blood pressure and tiredness)
Chance of dying within 3 months after treatment	Probably no additional risk of dying[c]	1.3%–1.7%	Unknown, but probably less than with surgery	Probably no additional risk of dying[c]
Chance of experiencing uncontrollable urine leakage (incontinence) as a result of the treatment	None	0.6%–1.2%	None reported	None
Need for future prostate surgery	Not well known; about 7%–55% at 3–5 years	2%–22% at 5–8 years	Not well known about 9%–35% at 1 year	Unknown

	Probably no additional risk.[d]	3%–35% (probably 5%–10% in men functioning entirely normal before surgery)	Unknown, but probably uncommon	Probably no additional risk.[d,e]
Chance of experiencing the inability to get an erection (impotence) as a result of the treatment				
Number of days lost from work or usual activities during the first year of treatment	1 day	7–21 days	4 days	3.5 days

[a]The number of + symbols indicates the relative improvement you may expect from each treatment.
[b]Most of the time these will not be severe, but 20% of the time they will be quite bothersome to you.
[c]The likelihood of dying for a 67 year old man is 8 out of 1000 within a 3 month period.
[d]One out of 50 men at your age loses his ability to have erection during sex each year even without any treatment.
[e]Information on alpha blocker treatment is not available.

It was the intent of the AHCPR that a large technical document would be developed, with a much shorter form for the practicing physician. This would include any physician, such as urologists, internists, and family practitioners, dealing with patients having BPH. Furthermore, a different version would be prepared for the patient, explaining the relative harms and benefits of diagnostic and therapeutic modalities. This would include the balance sheet developed by the panel. The patient would actively be involved in making decisions as to what would be his medical care.

The BPH panel adopted Dr. Eddy's terminology as to the relative strengths of their recommendation (Eddy 1990).

1. A *standard* is when the health and economic consequences of an intervention are very well-known and there is unanimity among patients and physicians as to the desirability or undesirability of intervention. A standard, therefore, is what most of us must do in a given situation.
2. A *guideline* is when there is sufficient evidence as to the outcome of an intervention to allow meaningful decisions by patient and physician. However, it would not necessarily be unanimous among these individuals but rather the majority (i.e., 60% of physicans). In other words, a guideline is what most of us should do in a given situation; however, a different action could be done when justified.
3. An *option* is when the outcomes are not clear as to the harms and benefits nor is patient preference really known. The physician would be in a situation to then intervene.

In summary, a standard is something that must be done; a guideline is something that should be done; an option is something that can be done.

Finally, the policy should have three basic requirements: (1) accuracy, the scientific basis for recommendations should be accurately presented; (2) credibility, the guideline should be applicable to the real world of medicine for which it is intended; and (3) accountability, the basis for the recommendations should be clearly defined.

At this time, the guidelines, developed by the AHCPR's BPH panel are to be released within the next 2–3 months. They will be in the form of a draft for evaluation and critique by individual experts as well as the appropriate medical organizations and may well be changed in the next few months after it is released. Thus, the guidelines that I will discuss in the diagnosis and management of BPH must be considered my own views. However, many of these guidelines were adopted by the World Health Organization (WHO) in Paris in June 1991.

Indications for Prostatectomy

Lytton et al. (1968) estimated that the chance of a 40-year-old man having a prostatectomy in his lifetime was approximately 10%; however, Glynn et al. (1985) raised the estimate to 29%. McPherson et al. (1982) noted that the incidence of prostatectomy, per 100 000 population, was 264 in New England compared to 122 in

England. Wennberg and Gittelsohn (1982) noted marked variation in the incidence of transurethral prostatectomy (TUR-P) within the United States. These studies raised the question as to whether or not different criteria were used to select patients for surgery, not only internationally but also within the United States.

The most common way of treating patients with bladder outlet obstruction, secondary to BPH, has been a TUR-P. Today, it is one of the most common operations performed (350 000 in 1985). It was second only to cataract extraction as the most costly major operation under Medicare, accounting for 1.4% total of Medicare allowable charges (Holtgrewe 1991; Holtgreve et al. 1989). In 1987, a survey of urologists revealed that TUR-P accounted for 38% of their major operations (Holtgrewe et al. 1985). With the increasing size of the aging population, one would expect a further increase in the number of TUR-Ps performed with a corresponding impact on money spent for medical care. Although TUR-P has been associated with a low surgical mortality rate and a good outcome, the need to control rising medical costs has caused the government and the medical profession to reevaluate prostatectomy with respect to indications for therapeutic intervention and the long-term and short-term results. Furthermore, new modalities of therapy are being introduced, such as α-adrenergic blockers, ballon dilatation, and 5-α-reductase inhibitors. Due to the large numbers of TUR-Ps being done, their economic impact on monies available for medical care (4–5 billion dollars per year), the apparent variations on their incidence, and the increasing number of newer modalities of therapy, it was obvious that guidelines for the diagnosis and management of BPH would be appropriate.

Recognizing BPH as a significant problem, development of guidelines for its diagnosis and management was one of the first three recommendations of the AHCRP In addition, as mentioned above, the WHO, recognizing BPH as a worldwide health problem, held a consultation in Paris in June 1991. Guidelines were developed for diagnosis and management of patients with BPH which were quite similar to those being developed within the United States.

There are very few studies on the natural history of patients who are seen initially because of modest symptoms of prostatism without absolute indications for intervention (e.g., acute urinary retention). Ball et al. (1989), in following 97 patients over 5 years, found that patient symptoms were essentially the same in 52% and worse in only 16.5%. Urodynamic studies revealed little change in that particular group and only 1.6% developed retention. Conversely, Birkoff et al. (1976), in following 26 patients for 3 years, found 50%–70% deterioration in patient subjective symptoms and 71% deterioration in objective criteria. Acute urinary retention was unpredictable.

There are certain indications that have been accepted as standard in patients over the years by urologists (i.e., acute retention, significant residual urine, hematuria, recurrent infections, azotemia, and bladder stones). In the AUA Cooperative Study (Mebust et al. 1989), 27% patients had acute urinary retention as the primary indication for surgery. It is impossible to predict which patients with modest symptoms of prostatism (i.e., symptoms of bladder outlet obstruction and bladder hyperreflexia) subsequently will develop acute urinary retention. However, Breum et al. (1982) found that 90% of patients presenting with acute retention required surgery in 1 year and Craigen et al. (1969) found that 58% required surgery within 3 months. The unpredictability of acute urinary retention implies another mechanism rather than just an accumulative effect of the natural progression of BPH.

Recurrent gross hematuria has also been considered as indication for intervention and occurred in 12% patients in the Mebust study (Mebust et al. 1989). The exact pathophysiology of the hematuria, secondary to BPH, is unclear but can lead to significant complications for the patient (i.e., clot retention).

Recurrent preoperative infection has been considered as an absolute indication for intervention. Preoperative infection was found in 12% of the patients in the Mebust study (Mebust et al. 1989). However, the incidence of infection was significantly higher in the black population (21%). The incidence of preoperative infection has been reported to be from 8.6% (Hasner 1962) to 25% (Melchior et al. 1974). The source of the infection presumably involves the prostate and is possibly related to the presence of residual urine. However, the incidence of recurrence of infection is not necessarily related to the exact amount of residual urine. Azotemia (defined as a creatinine greater than 1.5 mg percent) is also another indication for intervention. The incidence was noted by Holtgrewe and Valk (1962) (7%), Melchior et al. (1974) (18%), and the Mebust Study (Melchior et al. 1989) (9%). In the Mebust study, the indication for TUR-P, because of azotemia, was 4.5%. In following a group of patients, it is impossible to predict which ones will develop azotemia. Patients usually will present with significant symptoms of prostatism and are found to be azotemic. Many patients presenting with azotemia will be improved with relief of their bladder outlet obstruction.

Although these absolute indications for intervention are not uncommon, the most common reason for patients to undergo a TUR-P is symptoms of bladder outlet obstruction (i.e., decreased force and caliber of the urinary stream, hesitancy, straining to void, etc.) and symptoms of bladder hyperreflexia (i.e., urinary urgency, frequency, and nocturia). Some 90% of the patients in the AUA Cooperative study (Melchior et al. 1989) had significant symptoms of prostatism; however, 70% had another indication. Symptoms will vary over time in a patient who has an obstructing prostate. Ball and Smith (1982) noted, in a series of patients that were followed conservatively for a 5 year period, that 31% had improvement in their symptoms. Further, it was noted by Abrams (1977), in studying the effect of candicidin on patients awaiting prostatectomy, that 45% of the placebo group were much improved symptomatically. Therefore, any intervention has a tremendous placebo effect on patients, as far as symptoms are concerned.

Attempts to quantify the severity of symptoms has been attempted by Madsen and Iversen (1983) and Boyarsky et al. (1977). The physician needs not only to understand the severity of patient symptoms, but also how much the symptoms are bothering the patient and affecting his quality of life. In 1990, the AUA began plans to initiate a national cooperative randomized study on the different therapeutic modalities used in treating BPH and to compare their outcomes. In order to assess the effect of therapy on the patient symptoms before and after treatment, a committee was asked to develop a questionnaire that would document the severity of patient symptoms and look at the impact on the patient's quality of life and how much his urologic symptoms were bothering him. Starting with over 70 questions, Barry et al. (1992) developed an instrument that could be self-administered and which contained seven questions related to the severity of symptoms (Fig. 2), seven questions related to how bothersome the symptoms were, and five questions relating to the quality of life. This symptom index was validated by using it with patients who were seeing a urologist because of symptoms of bladder outlet obstruction and comparing them to the younger population who had no known BPH. The scoring system was validated as to its ability to discriminate between those who did or did not have BPH, the test/retest reliability, and internal consistency. The AUA Symptom Scoring Index was also compared to the Madsen/Iversen and Boyarsky systems and found to have a reasonable correlation. The WHO, in 1991, adopted the AUA Severity Index Scoring Questionnaire and also selected one global question

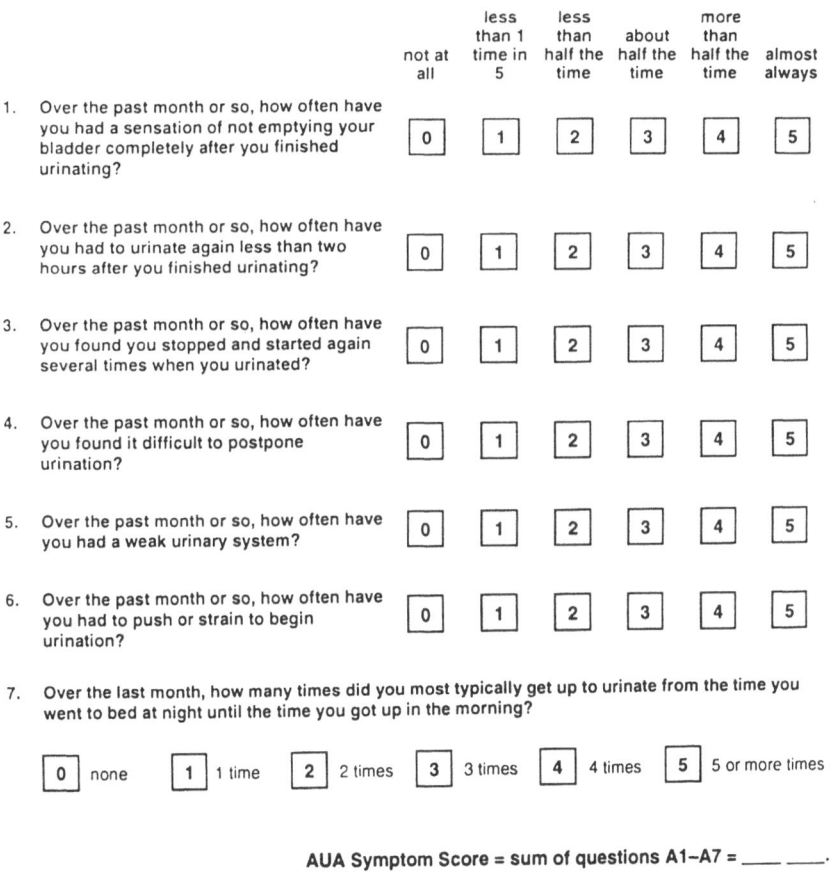

Fig. 2. American Urological Association (AUA) Symptom Scoring Index (Barry et al. 1992)

related to quality of life as affected by the urinary tract problems. The questionnaire has subsequently been disseminated as an instrument to evaluate BPH patients in France and other countries.

Initial Evaluation of Patients

Patients presenting with symptoms of bladder outlet obstruction, presumably secondary to BPH, must undergo an initial evaluation which would include a focused medical history. The focused medical history would include factors that might effect bladder function that would not be related to an obstructing prostate, such as medications affecting bladder function, possible neuropathies, and secondary to diabetes. A physical examination that would also focus on the genitourinary tract would be done, including a rectal examination which would provide information as to the size of the prostate. The latter is not related to the patient's symptoms but could be used to determine what type of intervention would be best suited for the patient. Furthermore, should the patient have findings suggestive of prostatic carcinoma, this would have to be evaluated. A urinalysis would be done as a general screen of the patient's kidney function and to rule out infection. A serum creatinine would also be employed to evaluate the patient's overall renal function. Using Dr. Eddy's terminology, these steps, in the initial evaluation, would be standard or something that must be done. Recently, prostate-specific antigen (PSA) has been used as a screening tool to rule out carcinoma of the prostate. While the specificity and sensitivity of PSA as a screening test is probably not good, it nevertheless is being used widely by many physicians. Since the exact role of PSA, as a screening tool, is yet to be determined, it could be included as an option in the initial evaluation of the patient.

Assuming that this initial evaluation indicates that the patient's symptoms are most likely secondary to an obstructing prostate, a more formal reassessment of symptom severity is undertaken. As noted above, the WHO recommended the AUA Symptom Scoring Severity Index and the one question on quality of life. However, at this time, the BPH Guidelines Panel will probably recommend just the seven questions regarding the severity of symptoms.

The objective symptom assessment would be done by any physician (urologist, general practitioner, internist, etc.) who is going to treat patients with BPH. Assuming the patient had mild symptoms and none of the absolute indications for intervention, he could simply be followed. The exact numerical score, which would differentiate between mild and moderate symptoms, has not been determined. However, one could imagine a patient scoring a 6 out of a possible 35 points on the AUA Severity Symptom Index and being assigned to, what has been called by Barry et al. (1988), as "watchful waiting." This should be considered a therapeutic approach, as the patient will need to return to the physician periodically for evaluation, which would probably include the assessment of patient symptoms, perhaps measurement of residual urine, urinalysis, and a focused physical examination. However, if the patient has moderate or severe symptoms, he might be offered watchful waiting, surgery, balloon dilatation, or medical therapy. Alternatively, diagnostic tests, based upon the physician and patient preference, would be undertaken to help determine if the patient really has an obstructing prostate. At this point, the patient should be carefully told the harms and benefits for each therapeutic and diagnostic modality. In developing guidelines, the AHCPR is including a consumer's guide, in addition to the physician's quick reference and the longer technical guideline.

In developing the practice policy for BPH, the panel had meticulously reviewed the world's literature and abstracted the raw data from appropriate papers. The harms and benefits of each therapeutic and diagnostic modality were combined using metanalysis, as described by Dr. Eddy (1992). The results were expressed in 5%–95% confidence profiles. This constituted a table of evidence which was then abstracted to present to the patient in the form of a balance sheet (Table 2). Since the relief of symptoms is probably the primary reason the patient seeks intervention, the balance sheet would carefully address symptomatic relief for each therapeutic modality. Using the confidence profiles, both the chance of improvement in the symptoms and the magnitude of the symptomatic improvement would be given to the patient. The chance for improvement of symptoms, for example, for TUR-P, range from 75% to 96% but had a four plus chance of improving the symptoms as far as magnitude of improvement as compared to balloon dilatation, for which the literature reveals the chance of improvement as approximately 59%–86% but with only a two plus magnitude of improvement.

The committee field-tested this balance sheet first by using it with a group of physicians who were not urologists but who were in the BPH group. They were given clinical scenarios as to the degree of symptoms involved, ranging from mild symptoms to acute urinary retention, and then asked which modality they would recommend for each scenario. The group of patients with BPH that were seeing urologists on the panel were then given the AUA Symptom Scoring Severity Index and asked to select which type of therapy they wished to have, not knowing how they had actually scored on the severity index. These scorings were used to group patients. In both groups, those with mild symptoms elected watchful waiting and those with severe symptoms (i.e., retention) selected more invasive therapy (i.e., TUR-P). Although the patients were somewhat more conservative than the physicians the trend was still the same. Both groups were asked which outcomes were important to them in making their decision. Relief of symptoms was considered by both groups as the most important outcome. The most significant risk or concern about intervention was the chance of developing urinary incontinence. Conversely, retrograde ejaculation played very little role in the decision making process. Using this information the balance sheet was modified to present information that the patients would wish to know, in a manner that was concise and clear. Using the Eddy terminology, the committee felt that offering treatment alternatives, in such a matter, should be considered a guideline or something that should be done.

In looking at treatment alternatives, the committee was struck by the fact that there are only two realistic alternatives: watchful waiting, which had been traditionally done, and surgery. The type of surgery is dependent upon the patient's prostate anatomy (i.e., large prostate, primary vesical neck contracture, etc.) and the surgeon's experience and skill. Medical therapy is certainly being used but many of the medications have not been specifically approved for the treatment of BPH (i.e., α-blockers). Other medical therapies (i.e., fenesteride) are becoming available; thus medical therapy would have to be considered as an option, depending upon the availability and government approval of the various medical modalities as it becomes available. Conversely, balloon dilatation, which had been approved by the Federal Drug Administration for treating BPH, was questioned by the panel as to its long-term efficacy. Also, in many areas of the country there is no reimbursement for balloon dilatation of the prostate. Therefore, this procedure would also have to be considered as an option, as far as presenting it to a patient.

Urologic Tests

Several tests have been used by urologists in evaluating patients with symptoms of BPH. Many of these were recommended as optional but not mandatory and others were not recommended as being used in the standard evaluation of patients.

Uroflowmetry

Perhaps the simplest and most noninvasive observation is urinary flow rate. However, this is dependent not only upon the degree of obstruction caused by the prostate but the contractility of the bladder. Nevertheless, most men with bladder outlet obstruction from BPH have an altered flow pattern compared to the normal. Siroky et al. (1979) developed a nomogram for average and peak flow rate adjusted for initial bladder volume. It was suggested that a patient whose flow rate was greater than -2 standard deviations from the mean was definitely obstructed. Drach et al. (1982) developed a nomogram adjusted for peak flow rate, taking into consideration the volume voided and adjusted for the age of the patient. Using this nomogram, an adjusted peak flow rate of less than 16 ml or greater than -1.3 standard deviations was considered suspicious for bladder outlet obstruction. The panel felt that uroflowmetry, adjusted for volume voided, could be useful in identifying patients with symptoms of prostatism because it would identify those with maximum flow rates that are not markedly diminished. These patients would benefit from pressure flow studies to confirm obstruction before therapy is carried out.

Pressure Flow Studies

These are studies in which the urinary flow rate is compared to the pressure generated within the bladder as the patient voids. The pressure in the bladder is determined by taking into consideration that contributed by intraabdominal pressure as one strains to void. These studies would not be used routinely in those patients who have usual symptoms and findings of prostatism. However, in those patients with an unusual history, physical findings, or objectives parameters, where the diagnosis is unclear, a pressure flow must be done. Furthermore, pressure flow studies are not readily available to all urologists. They are also dependent upon the skill and knowledge of the individual performing the test and it can be difficult to get test/retest reliability. The committee recommends pressure flow studies as an option.

Postvoid Residual Urine

Significance of residual urine is difficult to determine. It would seem logical that the greater the amount of residual urine, the greater the indication of bladder decompensation. There is very little data in the literature concerning postvoided residual urine. Hinman (1983) noted that over time, postvoided residual urine seemed to increase in those with an obstructing BPH. However, we do not know the amount of residual urine beyond which the patient will experience irreversible damage to his bladder from the obstruction caused by high-pressure voiding associated with an obstructing prostate. Therefore, postvoid residual has not been shown to be useful in predicting the need for or response to treatment. It is poorly reproducible for any given patient. However, for patients who are being followed with nonsurgical treatments, it is a technique to assess their status. Therefore, it is an option for the physician to use in monitoring patients. It should be done as noninvasively as possible. Roehrborn et al. (1986) found that transabdominal ultrasonography proved to be the least invasive and a sufficiently accurate method for determination of residual urine in men with symptoms of prostatism.

Tests Not Recommended as a Routine for Patient Evaluation

Upper tract imaging, by intravenous urography or ultrasound, has been used by many urologist in evaluating their patients with symptoms of bladder outlet obstruction secondary to BPH. In 1978, Greene stated that "excretory urography yields invaluable information concerning the upper tract in candidates for transurethral resection of the prostate. This examination not only detects significant renal and vesicle disease but more pertinent to the discussion, shows evidence of prostatic hyperplasia and sequela." The urologist is concerned that an occult renal cell carcinoma and hydronephrosis, secondary to obstruction, might be missed. The urologist has felt that information about the size of the prostate, the degree of bladder trabeculation, and the amount of residual urine could be obtained. Actually, using intravenous urography to determine residual urine is quite inaccurate. In an AUA survey by Holtgrewe et al. (1989), 73% of urologists routinely performed intravenous urography prior to TUR-P. The annual cost for such an examination would be somewhere between 66 million and one billion dollars per year. Ultrasonography would result in similar costs.

The committee evaluated 20 intravenous urography studies and nine sonography studies done on over 6000 patients with BPH. Depending upon the modality of evaluation, intravenous urography or sonography determined an incidence of renal cell carcinoma in the study population ranging from 0.18% to 0.56% which is similar to autopsy studies. It is highly unlikely that renal cell carcinoma is higher in the BPH population. Therefore, upper tract imaging is a poor screening test for renal cell carcinoma.

Conversely, there are harms that can be associated with intravenous urography, i.e., irradiation effects and the adverse effect of the contrast material used. Therefore, the committee did not feel that upper tract imaging should be used routine in patients with BPH but rather reserved for those patients who have a history of hematuria, urinary tract infection, renal insufficiency, refractory urinary retention, previous urinary tract surgery, or history of urinary tract stones.

Filling Cystometry

Filling cystometry (CMG) can be a useful urodynamic tool in evaluating urologic patients. It provides information on compliance, the presence and threshold of involuntary bladder contractions, and bladder capacity; however, it is an invasive study. A significant number of patients do have uninhibited detrusor contractions when they have an obstructing prostate. These correlated quite nicely with the symptoms used to determine the irritative symptom score. Thus, CMGs really do not add much to the preoperative evaluation of the patient but can be used postoperatively in individual patients who fail to have relief of the irritative symptoms to guide future treatment. Therefore, it is not recommended as a routine method of evaluating patients prior to intervention. Conversely, a CMG may indicate the preoperative patient that has a significant bladder decompensation. However, it is impossible to predict whether removing of the obstructing prostate in a given patient with a decompensated bladder will permit him to void adequately with a minimal amount of residual urine.

Cystoscopy

Cystoscopy is usually performed in the operating room prior to undertaking the surgical procedure. Therefore, it is not recommended as a routine office procedure in evaluating patients with obstructing BPH. Rather, it should be reserved for special situations in the preoperative setting. If the physician is unclear as to the exact diagnosis causing the patient's symptoms (i.e., bladder carcinoma causing irritative symptoms) then cystoscopy prior to deciding on an intervention would be appropriate.

In those patients who clearly have obstructing BPH, preoperative cystoscopy may be necessary to allow the patient to participate in the treatment decision and, more importantly, to inform him as to what is the best surgical procedure for his particular anatomy. In those patients who have large glands (i.e., over 70 g), an open prostatectomy may be more advisable than a transurethral resection of the prostate. Here, the patient would be informed that he was undergoing an operation that required an incision in his abdomen as opposed to the transurethral approach. In those patients who have a small prostate with a high bladder neck or primary vesical neck contracture they might be informed that they would be undergoing a transurethral incision of the prostate. Here, the patient would be informed that an additional biopsy would be necessary to help determine the presence or absence of prostate cancer.

Patients with large median lobes are not candidates for balloon dilatation and if the condition is present, this procedure could obviously not be offered to the patient. Ultrasonography of the bladder and prostate can also give information as to the prostate size and configuration and may be selected by some urologists for these purposes.

The recommendations in the practice policy or guidelines, as developed by the BPH Panel, are summarized in Fig. 3. I should point out that this algorithm is only an initial draft and may well be modified. As this writing, it has not been released for outside review. However, it is presented as an example of the type of treatment algorithms that may well be included in all practice policies or diagnostic and treatment guidelines.

Summary

Recently, there has been an increased concern over the appropriateness of medical care, as reflected in the geographical differences in the incidence of the various procedures. The cost for surgical intervention in patients with BPH consumes a considerable amount of our health care dollars. Alternatively, less costly and less invasive methods have been developed in the past few years. With the uncertainty as to the appropriateness of medical care, the cost in health care dollars, and newer modalities becoming available whose role is unclear in the management of BPH, patient care policy or guidelines were clearly necessary. Stimulated by these concerns and by Congress establishing the AHCRP, which mandated to develop its own guidelines, the production of individual guidelines by many medical groups has increased. The AUA's practice policy for the diagnosis and management of BPH was one of the first guidelines selected by the AHCRP. Several organizations have looked at what are the attributes or qualities that would make up a good practice policy. The explicit technique, as described by Dr. David Eddy, has been adopted by many organizations, including the AHCRP's panel on BPH, whose initial recommendations, as presented in this chapter, basically mirror those recommended by the WHO in June 1991. In assessing information used in developing these guidelines, it has become apparent that there is a significant lack of information concerning both the natural history of BPH and the relative value of the various modalities available to diagnose and treat BPH. The need for outcomes research is one of the significant findings pointed out by those developing patient care policies or guidelines.

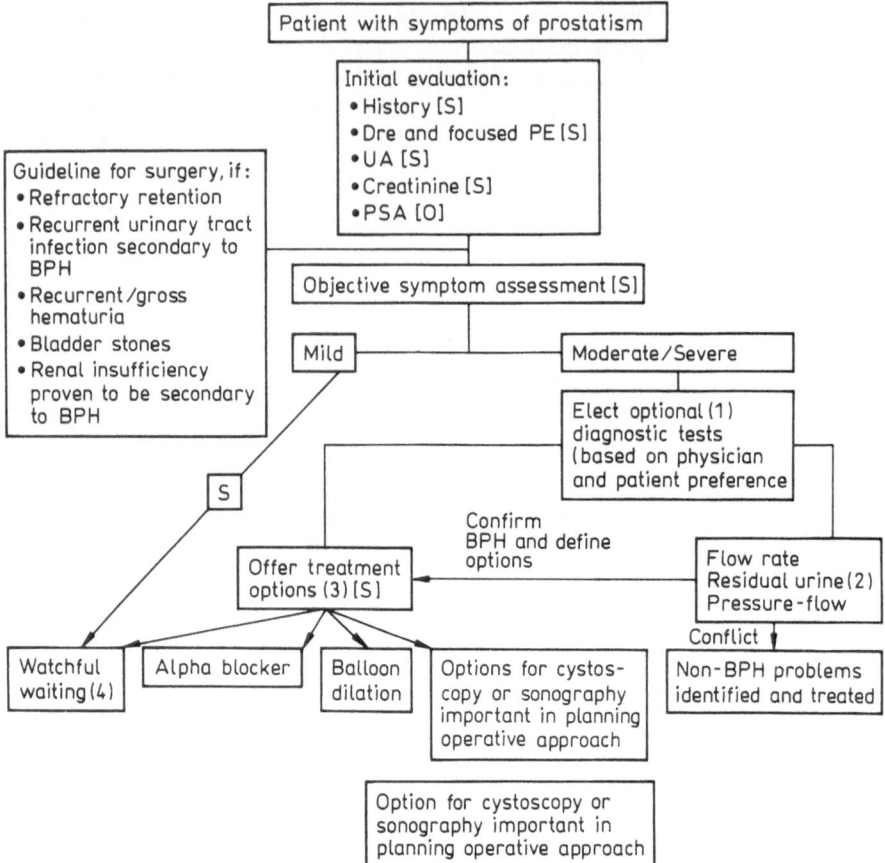

Fig. 3. Algorithm for the diagnosis and management of benign prostatic hyperplasia (BPH). Preliminary work of the Agency for Health Care Policy and Research (AHCPR) BPH panel. *S*, standard; *G*, guideline; *O*, option; *DRE*, digital rectal examination; *PE*, physical examination; *UA*, Urinanalysis; *PSA*, prostate-specific antigen

The recommendations, as presented here, undoubtedly will be changed and, in fact, will be scheduled for review on an annual basis. New information, diagnosis, and therapy will have to be considered as well as the impact of the current guidelines on the medical profession, their patients, and those bearing the costs of health care. It is hoped that the practice policies will improve the quality of medical care, but whether or not they will reduce the cost of medical care remains to be seen.

Practice policies or guidelines should be of help to practicing physician and not rigidly restrict him or her in the case of the individual patient. They must be developed by those involved in treating a specific disease; therefore, a multidiscipline approach is necessary. They must be clearly written and based on evidence that is explicitly stated and that can be carefully analyzed; the rationale for the recommendations must be understood. Formal rigorously constructed guidelines may have a significant impact upon medical practice now and in the future and must be constructed in good faith, keeping in mind that the ultimate application is to the patient's well-being.

References

Abrams PH (1977) A double-blind trial of the effects of candicidin on patients with benign prostatic hypertrophy. Br J Urol 49:67–71

Ball AJ et al. (1989) The natural history of untreated prostatism. Br J Urol 53:613

Ball AJ, Smith PJB (1982) The long-term effects of prostatectomy: a uroflowmetric analysis. J Urol 128(3):538–540

Barry MJ et al. (1992) The American Urological Association's symptom index for benign prostatic hyperplasia. J Urol (to be published)

Barry MJ et al. (1988) Watchful waiting versus immediate transurethral resection for symptomatic prostatism: the importance of patients preferences. JAMA 259:3010–3017

Birkhoff JD et al. (1976) Natural history or benign prostatic hypertrophy and acute urinary retention. Urology 7:48–52.

Boyarsky S et al. (1977) A new look at bladder neck obstruction by the Food and Drug Administration: guidelines for investigation of benign prostatic hypertrophy. Trans Am Assoc Genitourin Surg 68:29–32

Breum L et al. (1982) Significance of acute urinary retention due to infravesical obstruction. Scand J Urol Nephrol 16:21

Craigen AA et al. (1969) Natural history of prostatic obstruction. J R Coll Gen Pract 18:226–232

Drach GW et al. (1982) A method of adjustment of male peak urinary flow rate for varying age and volume voided. J Urol 128:960

Eddy DM (1990) Clinical decision making: from theory to practice – designing a practice policy standards, guidelines, and options. JAMA 263 (22):3077–3084

Eddy DM (1990) Guidelines for policy statements: the explicit approach. JAMA 263:2239

Eddy DM (1992) A manual for assessing health practices and designing practice policies. (In collaboration with the Council of Medical Specialties Societies Task Force on Practice Policies.) American College of Physicians, Philadelphia

Field MJ, Lohr KN (eds) (1990) directions for a new program. Clinical practice guidelines: National Academy, Washington DC, 52

Glynn RJ et al. (1985) The development of benign prostatic hyperplasia among volunteers in the normative aging study. Am J Epidemiol 121:78

Greene LF (1978) Selecting patients for transurethral prostatic resection. Geriatrics 33 (5):55–60

Greenspan AM et al. (1988) The incidence of unwarranted implantation of permanent cardiac pacemakers in a large medical population. N Engl J Med 318:158–163

Guidelines for permanent cardiac pacemaker implantation (1964) A report of the Joint American College of Cardiology/American Heart Association Task Force on Assessment of Cardiovascular Procedures (Subcommittee on Pacemaker Implantation). J Am Coll Cardiol 4:434–442

Hasner E (1962) Prostatic urinary infection. Acta Chir Scand [Suppl] 285:1–40

Hinman F Jr. (1983) Residual urine. Measurement and influence in management of obstruction. In: Hinman F Jr (ed) Benign Prostatic Hypertrophy. Springer, Berlin Heidelberg New York, pp 589–596

Holtgrewe HL (1991) Outcomes research and BPH, new concepts for deciding therapy. AUA Update Series, vol 10, lesson 20

Holtgrewe HL, Valk WL (1962) Factors influencing the mortality and morbidity of transurethral prostatectomy: a study of 2,015 cases. J Urol 87:450–459

Holtgrewe HL et al. (1989) Transurethral prostatectomy: practice aspects of the dominant operation in American urology. J Urol 141:248–253

Kelly JT, Kellie SE (1990) Appropriateness of medical care. Arch Pathol Lab Med 114:1119–1121

Lytton B et al. (1968) The incidence of benign prostatic obstruction. J Urol 99:639

Madsen PO, Iversen P (1983) A point system for selecting operative candidates. In: Hinman F Jr (ed) Benign Prostatic Hypertrophy. Springer, Berlin Heidelberg New York, pp 763–765

McPherson K et al. (1982) Small-area variations in the use of common surgical procedures: an international comparison of New England, England, and Norway. N Engl J Med 307:1310–1314

Mebust WK et al. (1989) Transurethral prostatectomy: immediate and postoperative complications. A cooperative study of thirteen participating institutions evaluating 3,885 patients. J Urol 141:243–247

Melchior J et al. (1974) Transurethral prostatectomy: computerized analysis of 2,223 consecutive cases. J Urol 112:634–642

Roehrborn CG et al. (1986) The role of transabdominal ultrasound in the pre-operative evaluation of patients with benign prostatic hypertrophy. J Urol 135:1190–1193

Siroky MB et al. (1979) The flow rate nomogram: I. Development. J Urol 122:665

Wennberg JE, Gittelsohn AM (1982) Variations in medical care among small areas. Sci Am 246:120–134

Assessing Treatment Results for Benign Prostatic Hyperplasia

A.J.Wein

Introduction

Nowhere in urology has the philosophy of treatment for a particular disease, or the list of options for treatment, changed so markedly over a short period of time as it has for benign prostatic hyperplasia (BPH). In 1985, in the second tome on BPH published by the National Institutes of Health (NIH), following an NIH sponsored conference on the subject, Frank Hinman, Jr. expressed the prevailing philosophy, at least among urologists, regarding the treatment of BPH: "Men will choose between continuing medical therapy for the rest of their lives or having a one time operation" (Hinman 1985). At that time, a short 7 years ago, the "medical therapy" consisted only of side effect producing means of decreasing serum testosterone or interfering with its action and nonselective α-adrenergic blockade. A tabulation of the treatment options for BPH now available is seen in Table 1, a list that will probably be incomplete by the time of publication of this volume. Lest one think this is a "pie in the sky" list, only two of these options (growth factor inhibitor and pyrotherapy) could be listed as laboratory, experimental, or theoretical considerations, while the rest are in fact real and available options, most of which are being vigorously pursued by one or another commercial company. At the 1992 meeting of the American Urological Association (AUA), there were two courses on balloon dilatation, one course on the pharmacology of BPH, one course on nonsurgical management of BPH, one course on new nonmedical trends in the management of BPH, and one course on hyperthermia!

The epidemiologic aspects of BPH are well covered elsewhere in this volume. It is agreed that between 400 000 and 450 000 prostatectomies are done yearly in the United States for what is originally diagnosed as benign prostatic disease. The total costs of prostatectomy for benign disease include not only surgical fees and hospitalization costs, but the costs of preoperative evaluation, lost productivity time, the treatment of complications, and similar considerations for reoperations. These costs account for a significant percentage of the American health care dollar. Added to these financial considerations have been three additional forces that have combined to produce great skepticism regarding aggressive answers to the pertinent questions of: Who will benefit from treatment of BPH? What kind of treatment is "best", considering cost, benefit, and risk? These forces are: (1) the recent emphasis on research with regard to long-term effectiveness and outcome of various medical procedures and practices (see Greenfield 1989), (2) the suggestion that the overall

Table 1. Treatment options for benign prostatic hyperplasia

Observation (watchful waiting)

Pharmacologic
  Bulk reducing
    Estrogen
    Luteinizing hormone releasing hormone (LHRH) agonist
    Antiandrogen
    5-α Reductase inhibitor (2)
    Aromatase inhibitor
    Growth factor inhibitor
  Tone reducing
    α-1-Adrenergic antagonist (6)

Surgical/mechanical
  Intraurethral stent (5)
  Balloon dilatation (5)
  Transrectal microwave hyperthermia (3)
  Transurethral microwave hyperthermia (2)
  Transurethral microwave thermotherapy (5)
  Focused extracorporal ultrasonic pyrotherapy (1)
  Laser prostatectomy (otomy) (2)
  Transurethral ultrasonic aspiration of the prostate
  Transurethral incision of the prostate/bladder neck
  Transurethral prostatectomy
  Open prostatectomy

The numbers in parentheses refer to the number of accepted podium or poster presentations at the 1992 meeting of the American Urological Association, Inc. on those particular modalities for the treatment of BPH or prostatitis.

outcome following transurethral prostatectomy is definitely not as favorable as hitherto assumed (see Roos et al. 1989), and (3) suggestions that, except in cases of severe symptomatology, urinary retention, upper tract deterioration, bladder calculi, and hematuria, prostatectomy may offer far fewer advantages over observation (watchful waiting) than previously assumed (Barry et al. 1988; Flower et al. 1988).

The specific purpose of this chapter is to discuss general and specific principles for the evaluation of the results of treatment of BPH. For the medical public, and for the general public as well, it is obvious that global terms such as "improvement" or "success" are no longer adequate. Much of the justification for surgical treatment of BPH was based on the fact that, as well as symptom relief, the procedure provided prophylaxis against the consequences of bladder outlet obstruction, and these consequences included detrusor decompensation, urinary retention, upper tract damage, azotemia, bleeding, and the progression of irritative/obstructive symptomatology. In addition, a commonly held belief amongst urologists seems to be that the longer symptoms persisted, or were allowed to progress, the less reversible they were. Some of these issues lend themselves to qualitative analysis, fewer to quantitative analysis, and some not at all. This chapter will concentrate mostly on parameters that are evaluable, recognizing that their significance to the patient and to the physician may be different. Financial considerations, immediate and delayed, will not be considered. Some general comments about prospective study design will be included.

General Considerations

Initial Considerations

Although an increasing number of clinical trials are of high quality, many still contain deficiencies of design, conduct, analysis, or presentation of results. Some qualify as only "pilot studies" in which a group, generally small, of selected patients are asked to undergo a new treatment. Those treated are generally coached as to the results to be expected. The treatment is not compared to either placebo or any other standard or nonstandard treatment except on the basis of historical results, and the best of these may not be chosen. Such a study generally serves only as a preliminary investigation, yielding information as to: (a) whether a particular treatment may have some value, (b) if so, over what period of time it should be studied to observe the maximum effect, and (c) what side effects may be expected. Such a study will also give statisticians some idea as to how many patients will in fact be necessary to properly investigate the treatment and compare it to others or to placebo. General criteria for an ideal clinical trial of a pharmacologic agent have long been available (Fingl and Woodbury 1975) and have been applied to BPH (Wein 1983; Heyns and deKlerk 1989). Such criteria, which can also be applied to procedures, include: a lack of bias, an adequate number of subjects, appropriate and sensitive methods of evaluation, double-blind conditions with a placebo, and statistical validation.

Bias Elimination

This generally does not constitute a problem. However, unconscious bias can occur, either in the assignment of patients to a particular treatment group or in the assessment of responses. Randomized, prospective, double-blind studies (see below) virtually eliminate this as a potential problem. If a study is not or cannot be randomized and/or double-blinded, the validity of the results can be considerably increased if the assessments are done by individuals other than those who assigned the patients to the treatment groups or/and who carried out the treatment.

Sample Size

Three primary considerations are relevant to sample size (Friedman et al. 1981): (1) the natural history of the condition under study, (2) the magnitude of difference expected as a result of the therapeutic intervention, and (3) the desired level of statistical significance. The theoretical and practical considerations relevant to sample size should be carefully considered with the aid of a statistician. The statistician must be aware of the type of data that will be generated and the magnitude of change to be expected. Otherwise, a given study may lack the ability to detect clinically important effects of significant magnitude or may overestimate them.

Appropriate and Sensitive Parameters of Evalution

Ideally, methods of evaluation will yield objective data in a form that can be easily analyzed statistically. Subjective data (e.g., symptoms) are generally difficult to quantify and analyze. Most symptoms defy exact quantitation and it is necessary to attach artifical grades to the severity of various symptoms and analyze changes in these. Although a symptom score (Tables 2–4 and Fig. 2 in Mebust, this volume) is a very logical and excellent idea, it is necessary, when dealing with small but statistically significant differences in such scores after treatment, to appreciate exactly what the symptomatic changes have been. Otherwise, the therapeutic efficacy of the treatment under consideration may in fact be overstated. Symptom scores, however, generally do not take into consideration what actually brought the patient to the doctor. Similarly, they do not take into consideration the effects of a given condition and its symptomatology or of an individual symptom on the patient's activities of daily living or overall quality of life. In other words, it is possible to favorably

Table 2. Symptom severity table (after Boyarsky et al. 1977)

Symptom	0	1	2	3
Nocturia	0	1	2–3	>4
Daytime frequency	1–4	5–7	8–12	>13
Hesitancy	<20%	20%–50%	50%–99% up to 1′	100% >1′
Intermittency	<20%	20%–50%	50%–99% up to 1′	100% >1′
Terminal dribbling	<20%	20%–50%	50%–99%	100% or >1′ or Wets Clothing
Urgency	0	Occasional	>50% May rarely lose urine	100% Sometimes loses urine
Impairment of stream	0	Impaired trajectory	Most of time size and force restricted	Great effort to urinate; interrupts stream
Dysuria	0	Occasional burning	>50% burning	Frequent and painful burning
Sensation of incomplete voiding	0	Occasional	>50%	Constant and urgent sensation; no relief on voiding

Table 3. Symptom score sheet (after Madsen and Iversen 1983)

Symptom	0	1	2	3	4
Stream	Normal	Variable		Weak	Dribbling
Voiding	No strain		Abdominal strain or Crede		
Hesitancy	None			Yes	
Intermittency	None			Yes	
Bladder emptying	Don't know	Variable	Incomplete	Single retention	Repeated retention
Incontinence			Yes (including terminal dribbling)		
Urge	None	Mild	Moderate	Severe (incontinence)	
Nocturia	0–1	2	3–4	>4	
Diuria	q>3h	q 2–3h	q 1–2h	q<1h	

Table 4. AUA quality of life assessment

	Delighted	Pleased	Mostly satisfied	Mixed about equally satisfied and dissatisfied	Mostly dissatisfied	Unhappy	Terrible
If you were to spend the rest of your life with your urinary condition just the way it is now, how would feel about that?	0	1	2	3	4	5	6

Quality of life assessment index L=

affect a symptom score without significantly affecting the actual complaint that prompted the patient to seek treatment. It is also possible to favorably affect the symptom responsible for the status change prompting treatment without significantly affecting an overall symptom score. An adequate protocol must also include a method for validation of a symptom score. In other words, if symptom status is derived primarily from patient generated forms, there must be a mechanism to show that these are in fact consistent with what would be obtained by an objective reporter questioning the patient.

Complications, including the necessity for retreatment, must also be considered. Some, such as the incidence of retrograde ejaculation, are relatively easy to quantify; others, such as decreased potency, are not. Complications must be assessed, furthermore, not only as to their incidence, but also as to their effect on overall life quality and activity.

Properly chosen urodynamic studies seem to be, at first glance, an obvious answer for an appropriate, sensitive, and objective method of evaluation of a given treatment for BPH. However, there is considerable disagreement as to what constitutes appropriate urodynamic criteria by which to measure the response of BPH to treatment. Most workers would agree that flowmetry is the most useful and reliable objective parameter by which to judge the success of treatment of bladder outlet obstruction. However, even relative to flowmetry, there are considerable disagreements as to: (a) what constitutes the most significant flowmetry parameter (mean vs peak flow, e.g.), (b) what constitutes a significant change, (c) the relationship between rate(s) and volume voided or total bladder volume and how to adjust for this statistically, (d) whether flowmetry should be totally noninvasive or in response to a standard filled volume through a catheter, and (e) the consistency of parameters in a given individual from one flow event to another.

Blind, Double-Blind, and Placebo-Controlled Studies

A prospectively randomized double-blind study is the ideal method to determine the clinical efficacy of a therapeutic intervention. Such a protocol virtually eliminates bias and, with an adequate sample size, ensures, as much as is possible, that the results obtained are due to factors other than simple sampling variability. A double-blind study is one in which the subject and the investigator are unaware of the identity of the treatment. This is ideally suited for the comparison of a drug with placebo or with another drug. It is difficult to utilize this methodology for an invasive therapeutic manipulation. Some interesting ideas have recently surfaced in this area, however, such as inserting a device without activating it. Dixon and Lepor (1991) carried out such a trial comparing the results of balloon dilatation and cystoscopy for the treatment of BPH. The negative conclusions they reached regarding this modality of treatment stand in stark contrast to other glowing reports of its efficacy. A similar trial of microwave thermotherapy is ongoing at the Mayo Clinic (D.M. Barrett 1992, personal communication).

There are obvious ethical considerations that pertain to the use of a placebo, particularly if there is a standard therapy that is clearly superior to placebo (Lebacqz 1979; Claridge 1983). However, it has long been recognized in protocols which use subjective criteria for assessment, that "improvement" may be expected in up to 35% of placebo-treated patients (Benson and Epstein 1976). This may be a result of true improvement that occurs in accordance with the natural history of the condition or it may be a result of the placebo effect itself. In general, the placebo effect can be boosted by a very positive, concerned, and enthusiastic attitude on the part of the treating physician, by the length of time spent with the patient, and by an intensive in-hospital type regimen (Benson and Epstein 1976; Lebacqz 1979). A patient in a placebo-controlled study must be told that the chances of receiving placebo are 50% and that a placebo is equivalent to no treatment at all. Provided the patient understands this and consents accordingly, provided a delay in currently accepted treatment is not hazardous to the patient's health, and provided the risks of the additional studies necessary as a consequence of the protocol are not unpleasant, hazardous, or unacceptable, no ethical problems are raised (Claridge 1983). If the subject is told and acknowledges that there is a 50% chance of receiving no treatment at all, this should decrease the placebo effect on subjective symptomatology and help to better define the true natural history of the condition under consideration. However, this also will decrease the number of patients willing to enter a particular study, especially if it is long-term. Unblinded studies, in which both the investigator and the patient know the treatment being received, are certainly easier to perform from the standpoint of patient recruitment, but unconscious bias and placebo effect are both significant problems. Single-blind studies with placebo are those in which only the investigator knows the therapy the subject receives. These are still subject to unconscious (investigator) bias.

In any type of study in which placebo is employed, it is obvious that the appearance and dose schedule must be the same as a drug under consideration. For a procedure, all steps up to and from actually applying the methodology should be identical. It would be ideal to eliminate any other factor that would enable the patient to ascertain whether or not placebo or medication/procedure is being received. Unfortunately, many clinically useful drugs have specific side effects and it may be impossible to build into a placebo the potential side effects of the therapeutic agent under consideration without making it something other than an inert compound. Institutional review boards generally require that the side effects of an agent, even in a double-blind placebo-controlled study, be detailed in the consent form. Although a perfectly sound ethical consideration, there is a question as to whether patients who receive active drug and who develop these side effects will be more subject to a positive placebo effect on the subjective symptomatology of the condition under consideration. For drug studies, to ensure statistical validity, some mechanism must exist to monitor patient compliance in taking medication or placebo. This generally consists of having the patient record the dose schedule and returning the unused medication at the termination of the study or at various points during the study when evaluation occurs. However, this does not guarantee that the patient has taken the missing drug. If a drug produces a measurable change in serum or a measurable change in some other status or function, this parameter can be measured to ensure that compliance has occurred.

Statistical vs Clinical Significance

Determination of the statistical significance of changes in an objective parameter is generally not a problem in a placebo-controlled study. Existence of a placebo group and the use of a double-blind methodology should eliminate any errors that might otherwise occur because of variability in results of a particular test, improvement that occurs as a result of the natural history of the disease, and statistical sampling. Subjective variables are difficult to quantify. Such items are often graded according to severity, and the resultant changes in grade subjected to analysis, either separately or in groups. Unless the changes are marked, this type of analysis has shortcomings. Adjacent categories or grades may exhibit only shades of difference that are not in fact clinically significant. Equally important, the concept of the most significant symptom, or what caused the patient to come to the physician in the first place, is absent from this type of analysis. Even more difficult to construct is an index that relates to the overall quality of life or what effect the symptoms have on the enjoyment or performance of the activities of daily living.

When considering objective changes, the concept of statistical vs clinical significance is paramount. For instance, an average increase in mean flow rate from 4 to 6 ml/s will, on average, represent a statistically significant change, as will a decrease in residual urine from 300 to 200 ml or a decrease in the number of daily episodes of urge incontinence from five to three. However, these changes may be less clinically significant for a given individual, especially if there are other forms of therapy which are capable of greater improvement or similar or slightly less improvement with fewer side effects. Investigators should point out differences between statistical improvement and what they consider to be clinically significant improvement. They should also compare these to the results of whatever the "gold standard" of treatment for that particular entity happens to be. In considering numerical differences, look for both absolute and percent change. Beware of investigators who preferentially express their data in terms of percent change rather than absolute values. Expression of data in this manner almost invariably makes treatment effects seem of greater magnitude than they actually are, further clouding the issue of real clinical significance.

Other Considerations

Crossover studies can be quite informative. Each subject receives one treatment initially and the placebo or alternative treatment during a second period of equal length. The order in which the treatments are given is randomized. This type of design ideally allows each subject to serve as his own control. However, a residual effect from one treatment can influence the effect of the succeeding treatment, and the duration of action of a given therapeutic effect must be considered. If this type of consideration represents a problem, there must be a "washout" period of sufficient duration between the first and second treatment period. A "lead-in" period may likewise be an extremely useful part of a given drug protocol. The lead-in period may simply be a period of baseline data collection without any treatment being administered, or it may include administration of a placebo to all patients, or it may be a combination (this seems ideal) of data collection during a period of no treatment followed by a period of placebo treatment to all patients. Most lead-in periods are 2–6 weeks, and the longer the lead-in period, the more information is generated regarding the natural history of the problem being studied and the magnitude of the placebo effect.

Entrance criteria for a study must be broad enough to permit most individuals to enter who actually have the problem being studied. However, the entrance criteria must exclude, as much as possible, patients with a condition that would favorably or unfavorably affect the results of treatment or would produce symptoms that might be confused with those of the disease under consideration. For BPH trials, it is generally agreed that patients with prior prostatic surgery, prostatic carcinoma, prostatitis, urethral stricture, bladder neck contracture, bladder stones, neuropathic dysfunction, and infectious or inflammatory disease of the lower urinary tract should ideally be excluded (Franks 1954; Wein 1983; Heyns and de Klerk). Likewise, certain categories of patients with various systemic diseases must be excluded as well as patients who are on, or subsequently placed on, other medications that may affect the clinical result or interact with a study drug. Data collection should be prospectively planned in such a way that all possible relevant variables are included. This permits prospective and retrospective stratification such that, if there are subgroups that may especially benefit from treatment or if there are in fact only certain subgroups that will benefit from treatment, these are readily identifiable.

Certain considerations are relevant in determining the minimal and maximal length of a study. Drugs must be considered not only according to their pharmacodynamic and pharmacokinetic characteristics, but also according to the type of physiologic effect they produce. In other words, if a drug reduces prostatic bulk by producing a metabolic change which begins fairly soon after the onset of medication, but the actual effect on prostatic bulk is exerted through an action on the epithelial component of the prostate that takes 3–6 months to become manifest, the study must continue at least for that period, especially if the effect is a gradual and progressive one. For instance, an α_1-adrenergic antagonist should exert some effects quite promptly, while an luteinizing hormone releasing hormone (LHRH) agonist will take 3–6 months or longer for the maximum effect to be seen. Similarly, a surgical procedure should produce some immediate results, but irritative side effects, which may mask the therapeutic effects, may take some time to resolve. The maximal positive effects of a surgical procedure may take months to become noticed, but it may take that long for certain complications to become manifest as well.

If a new treatment is being tested for a problem for which others are commonly used, it is of value to the clinician to compare the new modality not only to placebo or observation alone but to the gold standard of treatment for efficacy, selectivity, side effects, and cost. Finally, if a study is being carried out to determine the therapeutic efficacy of a noninvasive treatment for a condition that is generally treated by an invasive surgical procedure, it is critical to ask if the alternative changes the natural history of the disease as well as the invasive treatment does, and whether invasive treatment is eliminated or simply postponed. Conversely, however, one must be exceedingly careful to factor into an overall evaluation of a noninvasive vs an invasive treatment, the problems suffered by those unfortunate few who develop major adverse side effects following treatment – in the case of prostatic surgery, total or stress incontinence, impotence, retrograde ejaculation, bladder neck contracture, urethral stricture – and the necessity for retreatment or another operation. In other words, both short- and long-term "average" outcome should be considered.

Specific Considerations

Symptoms

Many parameters are available for study and evaluation in patients with BPH. Few physicians agree on the order of importance of these in assessing necessity for treatment and evaluating results of treatment. Consistent with the general principles previously expressed, a consideration of specific measurable variables in patients with BPH is in order, as these constitute the data base for the evaluation of the efficacy of any given treatment.

Symptoms have classically formed the initial data base on which to formulate evaluation of potential outlet obstruction, indications for surgery, and evaluation of treatment results. Symptoms are generally divided into so-called obstructive and irritative components. Obstructive symptoms occur during the emptying phase and include hesitancy, decreased stream, a feeling of incomplete emptying, straining to void, intermittency, postvoid dribbling, and urinary retention. These symptoms may reflect either bladder outlet obstruction or impaired detrusor contractility. Individuals who frequently void small volumes may also complain of some of these symptoms, simply because their voided volumes are so small. A patient with involuntary bladder contractions may likewise complain of "obstructive" symptoms when, after suppressing a small volume involuntary contraction, he rushes to the bathroom and finds himself unable to generate a voluntary contraction even after multiple attempts with straining, leaving him with the sense that he has at least intermittent marked difficulty initiating urination.

Irritative symptoms occur during the filling/storage phase of micturition and generally include increased daytime frequency, nocturia, urgency, and incontinence associated with involuntary bladder contractions. However, urgency, urge incontinence, and day and night frequency seem to occur most often in patients with BPH as a result of hyperactivity which has occurred in response to obstruction. Abrams (1985) cites the incidence of detrusor instability in patients with outlet obstruction secondary to prostatism as 53%–80%. The high reversal rate of this phenomenon following prostatectomy (reported as 45%–95%) certainly supports this association. Increased day and night frequency may also occur, however, secondary to poor emptying if a significant residual urine occurs, resulting in a decreased functional bladder capacity. Urgency may also occur because of a bladder which empties very poorly and is almost in "overflow" retention.

Symptom quantitation and meaningful comparison of symptoms before and after treatment are very difficult. To differentiate therapeutic from placebo effect, it is necessary to have a more exact symptom categorization than simply "better", "improved", "worse", or "no change." Two important facts bear emphasis: (1) the natural history of prostatism in some patients is indeed improvement and (2) there is a substantial placebo effect on subjective symptomatology For instance, Ball et al. (1981) looked at 107 of 318 original patients with prostatism who did not undergo elective surgery but were followed conservatively (no treatment) for 5 years. Ten of these reque has at least
intermittent marked difficulty initiating urination.

Irritative symptoms occur during the filling/storage phase of micturition and generally include increased daytime frequency, nocturia, urgency, and incontinence associated with involuntary bladder contractions. However, urgency, urge incontinence, and day and night frequency seem to occur most often in patients with BPH as a result of hyperactivity which has occurred in response to obstruction. Abr) studied the effect of candicidin on BPH in 62 patients awaiting prostatectomy. Of those who completed the study, 45% of the placebo group reported their symptoms "much improved" and an additional 17% reported them "slightly improved;" 38% reported "no change," and none reported worsening over a 6 month period. Using symptom scores, 34% reported improvement, 52% reported no change, and 14% actually worsened.

The concept of a symptom score or severity table for BPH was first developed by an ad hoc group formed by the Food and Drug Administration in 1975. The initial recommendations were published in 1977 (Boyarsky et al. 1977). Two of the first such symptom score formulations appear in Tables 2 and 3 (Boyarsky et al. 1977; Madsen and Iversen 1983). Investigators can and have played every game imaginable with such scoring tables, eliminating some symptoms and adding others, changing the weights and definitions of the severity of various symptoms, considering some symptoms separately, or dividing the symptoms into obstructive and irritative groups. For such a formulation to be produced, the patient can simply be asked to check an appropriate blank on a question and answer sheet or fill out a detailed diary or/and answer a series of verbal questions which will enable the investigator or a coordinator to generate a symptom score. As mentioned previously, there is generally no provision for considering specifically what actually changed most recently to bring the patient to the physician, what is in fact most annoying to him, what he wishes corrected most, or what effect the overall symptom complex, or any one symptom, has on his quality of life, general activities of daily living, or any activity in particular.

The AUA has, through its Measurement Committee, developed and validated a symptom score index (see Fig. 2 in Mebust, this volume, and Table 4) which has been adopted by the International Consensus Committee under the patronage of the World Health Organization (Mebust et al. 1991). This index takes into consideration somewhat the impact of the symptoms on overall quality of life. Validation in this setting means that the questions are clear and reliable: a patient answering the questions on a given day would answer them in the same way a week later (with no intervening treatment). Each patient is assigned a number for the symptom score (PSS) and for the quality of life assessment index (L). For the symptom score portion, 6–13 has been designated as "mild," 14–25 as "moderate," and 26–35 as "severe."

What constitutes a significant improvement in symptom score? The consensus of the Committee on Subjective Response, Objective Response, Impact on Quality of Life of the International Consultation on BPH (see Also et al. 1991) was that a reduction rate (of total score) of $\geq 50\%$ should be termed "remarkably effective", $\geq 25\%$ "effective," $<25\%$ "ineffective", and 20% "worsened."

Prostate Volume/Size/Weight

Prostate volume/size or weight are not necessarily related to obstruction or to the symptoms of prostatism, but changes are relevant for those types of treatment which nonsurgically reduce prostatic bulk. Digital rectal examination assesses primarily the posterior and lateral portions of the prostate, but such estimation of overall prostatic size is quite subjective, and it is difficult to assign an exact grading system which is universally agreed upon. Even with one examiner on different occasions, inconsistent readings may occur. Endoscopic evaluation of the degree of prostatic enlargement and obstruction is likewise highly subjective, and the reproducibility of estimates varies from examiner to examiner. Bladder neck to verumontanum distance seems to be the only objectively quantifiable parameter that relates to prostatic obstruction, although estimated prostatic weight and degree of lateral lobe occlusion have been cited as others (Andersen 1982). Certain parameters of urethral pressure profilometry (length and area under the curve) have proven reliable for the preoperative estimation of adenoma weight (Kitada and Ishisawa 1981). Ultrasonography is probably the best and most readily available reproducible form of total prostate size estimation; Peters and Walsh (1987) found an excellent correlation between sonographically estimated and pathologically measured prostatic weight after radical retropubic prostatectomy. CT scanning is an accurate method, but time-consuming, more expensive than ultrasound, and involves radiation exposure. Magnetic resonance imaging (MRI) can provide much more elegant and detailed images but at a greatly increased cost. MRI may hold the promise of being able to detect differential metabolic or size changes by zone, to distinguish periurethral from peripheral changes, and, perhaps, to differentiate epithelial from stromal change.

Endoscopic Findings

Endoscopic estimation of prostatic size has been mentioned with respect to size evaluation. Endoscopy has some value in excluding other pathologies, and its other main uses in the evaluation of prostatism are for the observation of trabeculation and for deciding whether an "open" prostatectomy would be necessary as opposed to a transurethral resection or incision. Although the prevailing sentiment regarding trabeculation is that it can occur in response to either obstruction, involuntary bladder contractions (probably because of accompanying pseudodyssynergia), or neurologic decentralization (Wein and Barrett 1988), Andersen (1982) found that trabeculation in his patients with prostatism was statistically related only to the urodynamic parameter of opening pressure. These comments about endoscopy are meant to apply only to its use in the evaluation of treatment results and not to its use in the overall assessment of the patient with voiding symptoms suggestive of BPH.

Flowmetry

There are significant disagreements regarding what constitutes an adequate urodynamic evaluation of prostatism and whether a urodynamically quantifiable definition of obstruction is necessary or desirable. This is not the place for a detailed treatise on the urodynamics of prostatism, but there are measurable urodynamic parameters, changes in which can indicate a favorable result, or a lack thereof, in response to treatment of BPH. Of all of these, uroflowmetry seems to excite the least controversy. Although diminished flow may be caused by either outlet obstruction or impairment of detrusor contractility and outlet obstruction may certainly exist in the presence of a normal flow, it is generally acknowledged that most men with significant bladder outlet obstruction do have a diminished flow rate and altered flow pattern (Blaivas 1989). Potential problems related to uroflow include the following: (1) many patients do not or will not void a sufficient volume for accurate measurements, (2) others void with an interrupted stream or with postvoid dribbling, which makes interpretation of the end point of micturition difficult, casting some element of subjectivity into the calculation of average flow rate, (3) some patients are unable to relax sufficiently to void in the same manner in which they would in the privacy of their own bathroom, and (4) a considerable discrepancy may exist between the first and subsequent measures of mean and peak flow.

  Since voiding events are invariably different from point to point in an individual's life, a variety of flow nomograms have been constructed to facilitate comparison of different flow events. Siroky et al. (1980) developed nomograms (Fig. 1) for average and maximum flow rates based upon flow rate measurements in a group of younger men, which were originally collected by Susset et al. (1973). According to these data the average and maximum flow rates depend upon initial bladder volume in a nonlinear fashion. The authors found relatively small variability in a single individual's flow rate over time and further concluded that urinary flow rate, when statistically related to initial bladder volume, could be used to estimate outflow resistance. Some 97.5% of normal men had flow rates consistently greater than -2 standard deviations at all points along the mean nomogram curve for average and maximum flow rate. The authors proposed that such nomograms

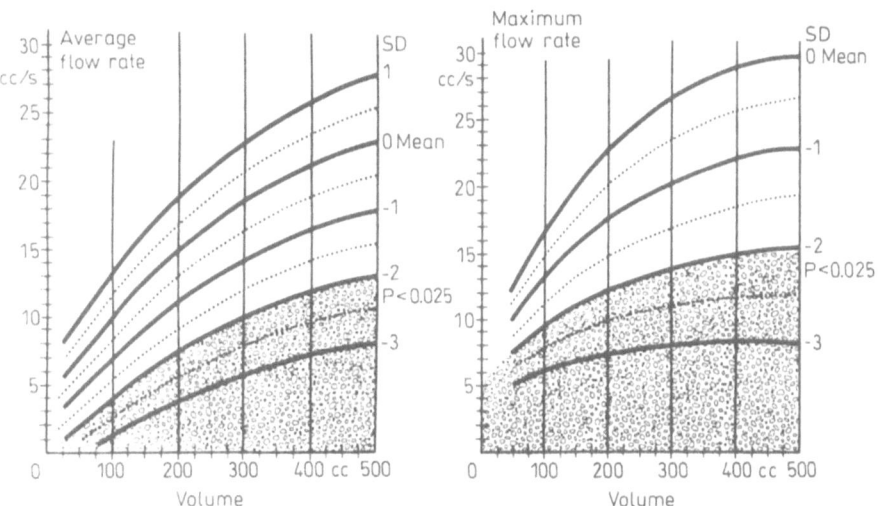

Fig. 1. Flow rate nomograms of Siroky et al. (1979, 1980) relating peak and average flow to intravesical (not voided) volume. The *shaded areas* represent flow rates highlly suggestive of outlet obstruction

could therefore be utilized to identify changes in outflow resistance after medical or surgical therapy. This is done by simply taking all measurements on one of the nomogram curves back to a standard bladder volume. The authors further concluded that consideration of voided volume rather than initial bladder volume resulted in a gross overestimate of an individual's voiding ability by an average of 2.1 standard deviations and that the smaller the voided volume in comparison to the initial bladder volume, the greater the overestimate. Drach et al. (1982) and Layton and Drach (1983) analyzed their flow data somewhat differently. They have stated that the adjusted peak flow rate is the most useful flow parameter to evaluate voiding dysfunction, and that this requires consideration of volume voided, rather than total bladder volume, and age. Their adjusted peak flow nomogram for males appears in Fig. 2. Using this nomogram, an adjusted peak flow rate of less than 16 ml/s or greater than 1.3 standard deviations below the mean is considered

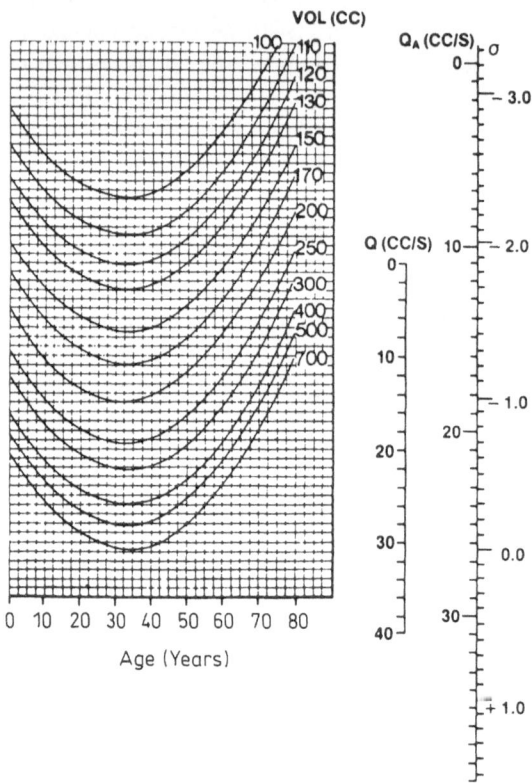

Fig. 2. Flow rate nomogram of Drach et al. (1982) relating peak flow, age, and voided volume. A perpendicular line is drawn upward from age until it intersects with curve for volume voided or is between two curves. Right angle line is then extended to right vertical axis of graph and point of intersection marked. Straight edge is used to join this point and observed peak flow (*Q*) on *middle scale*. Extension of this line intersects with right scale at point for adjusted peak flow rate (Qa) (*left side of scale*) or for standard deviation σ (*right side of scale*). An adjusted *Qa* of <16 ml/s or >1.3 standard deviations below the mean is very suspicious for obstruction

suspicious for bladder outlet obstruction. Although the details of these nomograms differ, and the authors' philosophies regarding important parameters likewise differ somewhat, each provides methodology for accurately comparing flow events at different times, which, after all, is the most important consideration in comparing flow data before and after treatment for BPH. It should be noted that there are many nomograms and tables of "acceptable flow rates" available for various age groups. Some individuals feel that the Siroky nomogram, the most commonly used in this country, overestimates peak and average flow rates for older males and therefore overestimates, according to their two standard deviation rule, the number of older males with bladder outlet obstruction. A recently published set of maximum and average urine flow rates in normal male and female populations (referred to as the Liverpool nomograms) confirmed that a certain amount of deterioration in male urinary flow rates occurs with age. As an example for comparison's sake, the Liverpool nomogram in "normal" men over the age of 50 sets a maximum urinary flow rate at a voided volume of 300 ml to be 21 ml/s at the 50th percentile and 11 ml/s at the 5th percentile. Corresponding average flow rates for these percentiles at this voided volume are 13 ml/sec and 8 ml/s (Haylen et al. 1989). It is doubtful that consistency will be achieved among flow nomogram makers. However, one of the systems supported by at least a portion of urodynamicists should be utilized for comparisons following treatment of BPH.

Residual Urine Volume

If significant residual urine is present, its reduction is an important parameter in the evaluation of results of treatment of BPH. Most patients with BPH (in my practice) have a minimal residual urine volume. For many or most with a significant residual it is impossible to differentiate deficient bladder contractility from outlet obstruction as the primary etiology without a pressure/flow study. Most would agree that the presence of a large residual urine volume ($\geq 150-200$ ml) reflects at least some bladder dysfunction, but it is difficult to correlate residual urine with either specific symptomatology or other urodynamic abnormalities (Bruskewitz et al. 1982; Hinman 1983). Insertion of a catheter is the most direct and accurate means of measuring residual urine volume, but, like a filled flow rate, this is invasive, causes discomfort, and may introduce infection. Noninvasive methods include isotope scanning and sonography. These are much more expensive and somewhat less accurate. Unfortunately for the BPH investigator, there may be a wide variation of residual urine volumes in an individual patient at different times (Bruskewitz et al. 1982; Hinman 1983; Birch et al. 1988).

Cystometry: Pressure/Flow Studies

Filling cystometry provides information on sensory integrity, compliance, the presence and threshold for involuntary bladder contractions and bladder capacity. Compliance is generally not affected in patients with only obstructive BPH, but, as mentioned previously, approximately 50% of such individuals will develop involuntary bladder contractions. Objective urodynamic documentation of the disappearance of this phenomenon following successful treatment of bladder outlet obstruction may be useful, as well as documentation of changes in bladder capacity. However, more important would be changes in concomitant symptomatology, such as day and night frequency and urgency.

On a logical basis, bladder outlet obstruction would seem to be defined, as Blaivas (1989) suggests, by the relationship between flow rate and detrusor contractility. Outlet obstruction is best characterized by a poor flow rate in the presence of a detrusor contraction of adequate force, duration, and speed. With obstruction, detrusor pressure during attempted voiding generally rises, flow rates generally fall, and the shape of the flow curve becomes more plateau than parabola-like. This is, however, marked disagreement about the utility of pressure/flow urodynamic measurements in the evaluation of suspected outlet obstruction and for the prediction of the success of treatment, at least by prostatectomy. Articles which best typify those which make an excellent case for the use of various types of pressure/flow studies, although some use other mathematical means to further complicate the relationship, include those of Abrams and Griffiths (1979), Coolsaet and Blok (1986), Jensen et al. (1988), Schafer et al. (1989), and Blaivas (1989). Equally forceful arguments against the utility of such measurements are made by Andersen (1982), Bruskewitz et al. (1982), and Graversen et al. (1989a,b). Jensen (1989) exhaustively reviewed the subject of urodynamic efficacy in the evaluation of elderly males with prostatism. One of the conclusions was that in this group interpretation of pressure/flow data using the nomogram of Abrams and Griffiths (1979) revealed a significantly better subjective outcome of surgery in patients classified as "obstructed" than those "unobstructed" (93.1% vs 77.8%). This technique is described in Fig. 3. Whether such measurements are necessary to evaluate the response of BPH to treatment and how much they add to the evaluation of the efficacy of a drug or procedure are issues that are as yet unsettled. Successful treatment of BPH by prostatectomy is generally correlated with a reduction in the detrusor pressure during an increased uroflow. Consideration of the entire pressure/flow plot as described by Abrams and Griffiths (1979) may in fact prove to be a more accurate and informative way of looking at this relationship. Other still more complicated ways of evaluating simultaneous flow and pressure may

---

Fig. 3. a Nomogram of maximum flow rate vs detrusor pressure at maximum flow. The *two lines* divide the figure into three zones: obstructed, equivocal, and unobstructed. A correction of 0.5 s is made for the time lag (Jensen 1989). By means of X-Y plots it is decided whether patients in the equivocal zone are obstructed (Abrams and Griffiths 1979). With no obstruction after a fast initial rise in flow rate the mean slope of the pressure/flow plot is <2 cm H_2O/ml s^{-1} and the pressure at the end of voiding <40 cm H_2O. Patients whose plots show a mean flow >2 cm H_2O/ml s^{-1} and with mean slope <2 cm H_2O/ml s^{-1} but with pressure at end of voiding >40 cm H_2O are classified as having obstruction. **b** X-Y plot indicating no obstruction. Plot is nearly horizontal (mean slope is small) and pressure ahead of voiding is low. **c** X-Y plot from a patient with obstruction. Plot is not horizontal and mean slope (after fast initial rise of flow rate) is large. This pattern plot is often curved so that the mean slope can be only roughly estimated. However, little ambiguity is present since the curvature helps to classify the pattern as obstructed. **d** X-Y plot indicating obstruction. Plot is nearly horizontal but pressure at end of voiding is high. (From Abrams and Griffiths 1979)

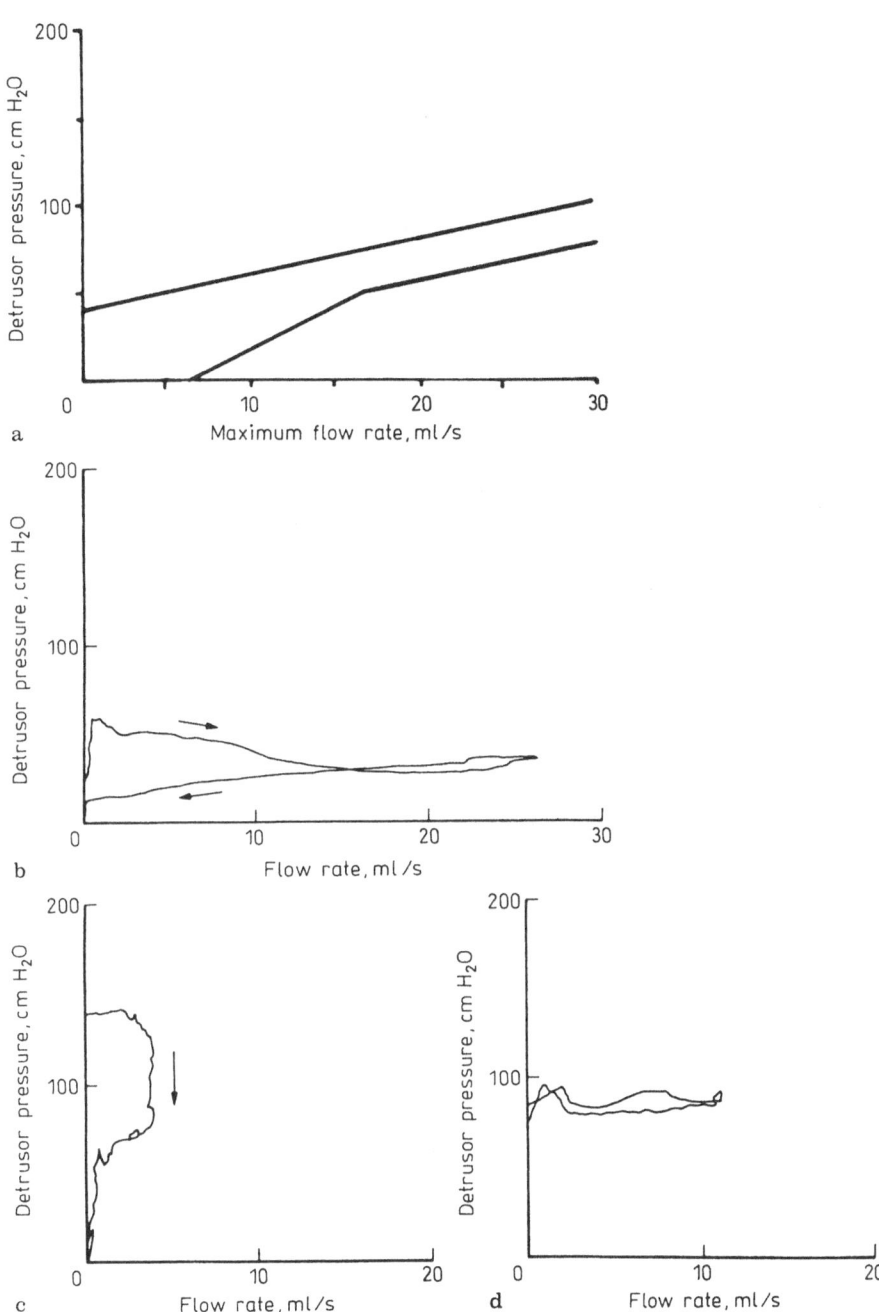

narrow further still the diagnostic "grey zone" between bladder outlet obstruction and decreased detrusor function and may permit a more precise way of assessing treatment response. It seems fair to say that, at this time, although this type of invasive study may be the most accurate in urodynamically describing response to treatment, it should be the last performed to complete the profile of action of a given drug or procedure on patients with BPH.

Symptomatic vs Urodynamic Improvement

There is one other consideration which should be mentioned and that is the seeming dissociation which may occur between symptomatic and urodynamic improvement. This has been most notable in data concerning some newer "make a hole" technologies and pharmacologic agents. The fact that symptomatic improvement occurs which is seemingly out of proportion to the amount of urodynamic improvement might in fact be assumed to indicate that a given treatment is not equal to the current "gold standard" of prostatectomy, or that the results will be of shorter duration. However, one important possibility to consider is that the actual symptoms of prostatism have much less to do with urodynamically defined obstruction than we think and that relief with these other types of treatment has to do more with the correction of some ill-defined mechanism within the prostatic urethra that is not directly related to the amount of mechanical obstruction. Alternatively, it may not be necessary to reduce outlet obstruction by an amount similar to prostatectomy to significantly improve symptomatology and prevent bladder or/and upper tract deterioration.

Complications

Although the occurrence of complications is factored into the issue of overall quality of life in assessing treatment results, specific problems bear special mention here since the gold standard of treatment for BPH has been surgery. In comparing outcome likelihoods from one treatment modality to another, comparable risks must be included for those problems associated with the gold standard. These include bleeding, transfusion, infection, retention, hyponatremia, urethral stricture, bladder neck contracture, stress incontinence, total incontinence, retrograde ejaculation, impotence, and death.

Summary

For years many have assumed that the symptoms of prostatism were due to obstruction, that it was necessary to overcorrect the obstruction to optimally relieve these symptoms (compare the prostatic fossa of a normal 18 year old male to one after prostatectomy), and that, if obstruction was not corrected, dire consequences would result in at least some of those affected. These could include detrusor decompensation, urinary retention, upper tract damage, infection, azotemia, symptoms irreversibility, and even death. Studies on the natural history of prostatism have shown, at least for the short term, that such consequences occur in a very small minority of patients. Recent studies on a variety of alternate technologies for the treatment of BPH, in addition, have shown acceptable or even equivalent (to prostatectomy) symptom relief, in short-term follow-up at least. Some method of comparison of the results of prostatectomy vs these alternate technologies vs watchful waiting (observation) is obviously necessary. This chapter has summarized some of the considerations relative to these assessments. Prospective application of such general and specific principles will ultimately allow us to pass valid judgment on treatment versus no treatment and on the merits of specific types of therapy. This would have undoubtedly pleased William Heberden, whose experience and common sense prompted his comment, "New medicines and new methods of cure always work miracles for a while" (Wein 1990).

References

Abrams PH (1977) A double blind trial of the effects of candicidin on patients with benign prostatic hypertropy. Br J Urol 53:613

Abrams P (1985) Detrusor instability and bladder outlet obstruction. Neurourol Urodyn 4:317

Abrams PH, Griffiths DJ (1979) The assessment of prostatic obstruction from urodynamic measurements and from residual urine. Br J Urol 51:129

Anderson JT (1982) Prostatism: clinical, radiologic and urodynamic aspects. Neurourol Urodyn 1:241

Aso Y, Boccon-Gibod L, Colais DaSilva F, Chaussy C, Fowler J, Homma Y, Legrain M, Moriyama N, Richard F, Tazaki H (1991) Subjective response, objective response impact on quality of life. In: Cockett A, Aso Y, Chatelain et al. (eds) Proceedings of the international consultation on BPH, Digital Print, Ivry/Seine, France, 1991, pp 87–90

Ball AJ, Feneley RCL, Abrams PH (1981) The natural history of untreated "prostatism". Br J Urol 53:613

Barry MJ, Mulley AG, Fowler FJ, Wennberg JW (1988) Watchful waiting versus immediate transurethral resection for symptomatic prostatism: the importance of patients' perferences. JAMA 259:2010

Benson H, Epstein MD (1976) The placebo effect. JAMA 232:1225

Birch NC, Hurst G, Doyle PT (1988) Serial residual volumes in men with prostatic hypertrophy. Br J Urol 62:571

Blaivas JG (1989) Evaluation of bladder outlet obstruction. In: Paulsen DF (ed) Prostatic disorders. Lea and Febiger, Philadelphia, pp 173–192

Boyarsky S, Jones G, Paulson DF, Prout GR Jr (1977) A new look at bladder neck obstruction by the food and drug administration: guidelines for investigation of benign prostatic hypertrophy. Trans Am Assoc Genitourin Surg 68:29

Bruskewitz RC, Iverson P, Madsen PO (1982) Value of postvoid residual urine determination in evaluation of prostatism. Urology 20:602

Bruskewitz R, Jensen KME, Iversen P, Madsen PO (1983) The relevance of minimum urethral resistance in prostatism. J Urol 129:769

Claridge M (1983) Assessment of medical treatment. In: Hinman F Jr (ed) Benign Prostatic Hypertrophy. Springer, Berlin, Heidelberg New York, pp 308–312

Coolsaet B, Blok C (1986) Detrusor properties related to prostatism. Neurourol Urodyn 5:435

Dixon CM, Lepor H (1991) Transurethral dilatation of the prostate. Probl Urol 5(3):463

Drach GW, Layton T, Bottaccini MR (1982) A method of adjustment of male peak urinary flow rate for varying age and volume voided. J Urol 128:960

Fingl E, Woodbury DM (1975) General principles. In: Goodman LS, Gilman A (eds) The pharmacologic basis of therapeutics. Macmillan, New York, pp 1–46

Fowler FJ, Wennberg JE, Timothy RP, Barry MJ, Mulley AG, Hanley D (1988) Symptom status and quality of life following prostatectomy. JAMA 259:3018

Franks LM (1954) Benign hyperplasia of prostate. Ann Roy Coll Surg 14:92

Friedman LM, Furberg CD, DeMetz DL (1981) Fundamentals of clinical trials. Wright, Boston, pp 69–88

Geller J, Nelson CG, Pilbert JD, Pratt C (1979) Effect of megestrol acetate on uroflow rates in patients with benign prostatic hypertrophy. Urology 14:467

Graversen PH, Gasser TC, Wasson JH, Hinman F Jr, Bruskewitz RC (1989a) Controversies about indications for transurethral resection of the prostate. J Urol 141:475

Graversen PH, Bruskewitz RC, Madsen PO (1989b) The predictive value of urodynamic investigations for results following prostatectomy. In: Paulson DF (ed) Prostatic disorders, Lea and Febiger, Philadelphia, pp 232–245

Greenfield S (1989) The state of outcome research: are we on target? NEJM 320:1142

Haylen BT, Sabby D, Sutherst JR, Frazer MI, West CR (1989) Maximum and average urine flow rates in normal male and female populations-the Liverpool nomograms. Br J Urol 64:30

Heyns CF, deKlerk DP (1989) Pharmaceutical management of benign prostatic hyperplasia. In: Paulson DF (ed) Prostatic disorders. Lea and Febiger, Philadelphia, pp 204–231

Hinman F Jr (1983) Residual urine: measurement and influence in management of obstruction. In: Hinman F Jr (ed) Benign Prostatic Hypertrophy. Springer, Berlin Heidelberg New York, pp 589–596

Hinman, F., Jr. (1985) Overview – basis for clinical management, BPH, vol 2, NIH Publ 87–2881, Bethesda, p 205

Jensen KME (1989) Clinical evaluation of routine urodynamic investigations in prostatism. Neurourol Urodyn 8:545

Jensen KME, Jorgensen JB, Magnesen P (1988) Urodynamics in prostatism: II. Prognostic value of pressure-flow study combined with stop-flow test. Scand J Urol Nephrol [Suppl] 114:72

Kitada S, Ishisawa N (1981) Urethral pressure profilometry in the prospective assessment for prostatectomy. J Urol 126:89

Layton TM, Drach GW (1983) Urinary flow rates: measurement and adjustment. In: Hinman F Jr (ed) Benign Prostatic Hypertrophy. Springer, Berlin Heidelberg New York, pp 524–527

Lebacqz K (1979) Controlled clinical trials: some ethical issues. Controlled Clin Trials 1:29

Lytton B, Emery JM, Howard BM (1968). The incidence of benign prostatic obstruction. J Urol 99:639

Madsen PO, Iversen P (1983) A point system for selecting operative candidates. In: Hinman F Jr (ed) Benign Prostatic Hypertrophy. Springer, Berlin Heidelberg New York, pp 763–765

Mebust W, Roizo R, Schroeder F, Villers A (1991) Correlations between pathology, clinical symptoms and the course of the disease. In: Cockett A, Aso Y, Chatelain B et al. (eds) Proceedings of the international consultation on BPH, digital print, Ivry/Seine, France, pp 53–62

Peters CA, Walsh PC (1987) The effect of naferelin acetate, a leutinizing hormone releasing hormone agonist on benign prostatic hyperplasia. NEJM 317:599

Roos NP, Wennberg JE, Malenka DJ, Fisher ES, McPherson K, Andersen TF, Cohen MM, Ramsey E (1989) Mortality and reoperation after open and transurethral resection of the prostate for benign prostatic hyperplasia. NEJM 320:1120

Schafer W, Rubben H, Noppeney R, Deutz FJ (1989) Obstructed and unobstructed prostatic obstruction: a plea for urodynamic objectivation of bladder outflow obstruction in benign prostatic hyperplasia. World J Urol 6: 198

Siroky MB, Olsson CA, Krane RJ (1979) The flow rate nomogram: I. Development. J Urol 122:665

Siroky MB, Olsson CA, Krane RJ (1980) The flow rate nomogram: II. Clinical correlations. J Urol 123:208

Susset JG, Picker P, Kretz M, Jorest R (1973) Critical evaluation of uroflometers and analysis of normal curves. J Urol 109:874

Wein AJ (1981) Where are we: clinical trials. In: Zinner NR, Sterling AR (eds) Female incontinence, Liss, New York, pp 39–43

Wein AJ (1983) Principles for evaluation of pharmacologic agents. In: Hinman F Jr (ed) Benign Prostatic Hypertrophy. Springer, Berlin Heidelberg New York, pp 414–418

Wein AJ (1990) Evaluation of treatment response to drugs in benign prostatic hyperplasia. Urol Clin North Am 17(3):631

Wein AJ, Barrett DM (1988) Voiding function and dysfunction: a logical and practical approach. Year Book Medical Publishers, Chicago, pp 278–280 a

Urodynamic Assessment of Benign Prostatic Hypertrophy

M.P.Sullivan and S.V.Yalla

Introduction

The primary goal of surgical treatment of benign prostatic hypertrophy (BPH) is the relief of bladder outlet obstruction. However, only 84% of those patients presenting with moderate symptoms of prostatism who are surgically treated will show symptomatic improvement (Lepor and Gilbert 1990). A recent study, which estimates that as many as 25% of prostatectomy patients may actually be unobstructed (Schäfer et al. 1988), underscores the value of an appropriate urodynamic evaluation that will provide objective indications for surgical intervention and predict favorable treatment outcomes. As the number of transurethral prostatectomies (TURPs) performed annually climbs over 500000, the potential for unnecessary or inadequate surgical procedures continues to rise at an alarming rate. Therefore, an accurate understanding of the mechanism responsible for BPH symptoms is essential for the appropriate management of the voiding dysfunction.

The glandular and stromal hyperplasia associated with BPH induces substantial increases in tissue volume and marked alterations in the geometry and architecture of the prostate gland. These anatomical changes may eventually progress to produce clinical symptoms of prostatic urethral dysfunction or prostatism. However, the mere presence of an enlarged prostate gland does not signify the inevitable emergence of clinical symptoms of bladder outlet obstruction. Often, concomitant prostatic pathology such as infarctions, prostatitis, or adenocarcinoma are responsible for precipitating the onset of prostatism. The pathologic structure of the lesion and the characteristics of the prostatic capsule may also influence the clinical progression of asymptomatic BPH to bladder outlet obstruction. Prostates with predominately fibromuscular components cause infravesical outlet obstruction by altering urethral compliance and impeding flow, although the glands may not appear enlarged on rectal and cystoscopic evaluation. The elastic properties of the surrounding prostatic capsule determine whether growth of BPH nodules results in either expansion of prostate tissue without compromising urethral opening or compression of the prostatic urethra.

The complex of obstructive (hesitancy, interrupted or decreased force of urinary stream, incomplete emptying, terminal dribbling) and irritative (frequency, nocturia, urgency) symptoms that are usually ascribed to BPH are not necessarily unique to bladder outlet obstruction. Particularly in the elderly patient group, the prevalence of comorbid disease such as myeloneuropathies secondary to disc disease, spondylosis, ischemic dysfunction resulting from peripheral vascular disease, diabetes, stroke, congestive heart failure, and peripheral edema may result in symptoms that mimic those of BPH. In our own recent studies, precise electrodiagnostic testing of this population has shown that covert and comorbid neurologic abnormalities can be identified in 83% of our elderly patients with prostatism (Dyro et al. 1992). The extent to which these neuropathologies contribute to symptoms of prostatism, however, remains unclear. Other sources of symptomatic voiding dysfunction that are not related to outlet obstruction include structural changes accompanying normal aging of the bladder and polypharmacia (the indulgence in various pharmacologic agents such as cholinergics, anticholinergics, calcium channel blockers, and cold remedies containing sympathomimetics). Because of the potential for these coexisting conditions in the elderly population, the underlying etiology of the prostatism symptoms or voiding dysfunction can often be multifactorial.

The diagnostic value of the prostatism symptom complex is sometimes problematic since these symptoms are not a necessary or even a specific indication of prostatic enlargement or outlet obstruction in the elderly male population. In fact, many of these symptoms are also observed in elderly females. Irritative symptoms such as frequency, nocturia, and urge are commonly attributed to detrusor instability (DI). Although DI is often associated with outlet obstruction and is observed in two thirds of patients presenting with prostatism (Anderson 1982), no correlation has been found between the presence of DI and prostate size (Cucchi 1980); furthermore, the degree of outlet obstruction does not portend the imminent development of DI (Jensen et al. 1988). Some irritative symptoms, instead of resulting from detrusor hyperactivity, may be precipitated by a large capacity, hypocontractile detrusor. In these patients, the incomplete emptying, which is responsible for the frequency of urination, may erroneously be ascribed to obstruction-related detrusor irritability. Irritative symptoms can also be caused by neurogenic detrusor hyperactivity, or more appropriately, detrusor hyperreflexia.

Similarly, the accurate diagnosis of obstructive voiding dysfunction using the obstructive symptom complex of prostatism is unreliable. These symptoms correlate poorly with the weight of prostate tissue resected at TURP (Jensen et al. 1983) and, in a significant percentage of patients, can be related to dysfunction of the detrusor in the absence of outlet obstruction (Coolsaet and Blok 1986). In addition, features that are conventionally considered to be unequivocal evidence of outlet obstruction – acute urinary retention (Klarskov et al. 1987) and postvoid residual volume (Turner-Warwick et al. 1973) – may well denote detrusor dysfunction rather than BPH. Therefore, symptoms of voiding dysfunction, either obstructive or irritative in nature, are highly nonspecific and do not necessarily indicate the underlying pathophysiology of the voiding dysfunction.

The fundamental aims of urodynamic evaluation in patients with prostatism symptoms are to: (a) characterize the functional behavior of the lower urinary tract; (b) correlate the lower urinary tract dysfunction with prostatic enlargement and obstruction; (c) confirm the presence of bladder outlet obstruction and identify its location; (d) assess the degree of prostatic urethral obstruction and predict its prognostic outcome; (e) evaluate the detrusor contractile efficiency; (f) identify subclinical neuropathic vesicourethral dysfunction mimicking or compounding prostatic obstruction and determine the extent of its contribution. This last point is particularly important in patients with overt neuropathology, such as diabetic autonomic neuropathy, stroke, Parkinsonism, and disc disease, who may also have prostatic enlargement. Detailed urodynamic studies in these patients may provide information regarding the contribution of the individual pathologies to the BPH symptoms.

Since conventional urologic evaluation of prostatism (patient symptoms, digital rectal exam, postvoid residual volume, intravenous pyelography, cystourethroscopy) cannot reliably or effectively assess outlet obstruction, further urodynamic evaluation is indispensable for the accurate diagnosis of vesicourethral dysfunctions. Many innovative urodynamic tests have been proposed to objectively characterize the detrusor contractile performance and the conduit properties of the bladder outlet. Although some of these may appear complex and cumbersome and technically difficult to perform, they are an essential component of the urologists' armamentarium in the assessment of functional abnormalities of micturition.

Urinary Flow Rate Measurements

The simplest screening device to assess outlet obstruction is the uroflowmeter. This diagnostic tool provides an inexpensive, cost-effective and noninvasive method of documenting urinary flow. Its routine usage in hospitals, outpatient clinics, and private offices allows physicians to follow the progression of a patient's pathology and evaluate the effectiveness of various treatment options.

Urinary flow rate is defined as the volume of urine collected over a given period of time and is usually expressed in milliliters per second. Several commercial uroflowmeters that are currently available measure urinary flow using one of the following methods: air displacement, volumetric, gravimetric, momentum flux, or electromagnetic measurement principles. With the exception of the electromagnetic flowmeters, most of these instruments operate by differentiating volume with respect to time and thus provide only an approximation of instantaneous flow rate. The patient is instructed to void into a flowmeter in a manner that is indicative of his usual voiding habits. To ensure reproducibility, additional flow curves may be required. Documentation of a patient's micturition pattern and measurements of maximum flow rate (Q_{max}) and voided volume provide the most useful parameters that can adequately characterize an individual's flow curve. Other descriptive parameters related to urinary flow that are used less frequently include the average flow rate, total voiding time, time to peak flow, and flow at 2 s.

Peak urinary flow rates greater than 15 ml/s are generally considered normal. The populations mean for Q_{max} is 26.3 cc/s for a 44 year old male who voids 326 ml (Layton and Drach 1983). The normal flow curve is characterized by a reasonably symmetrical bell-shaped pattern that rises steeply to peak flow rate within the first third of the total voiding time, similar to the curve shown in Fig. 1b. Following a period of relatively stable flow, the trace descends at a slower rate than the initial rise. Deviations from this typical flow shape can often signal potential dysfunctions. Irregular or interrupted uroflow patterns can be indicative of abdominal straining, sphincter contraction or even flow measurement artifacts, while "box-shaped" curves are often associated with urethral strictures. The uroflow patterns of patients with prostatic obstruction are typically characterized by continuous, elongated, and reduced flow curves in which the maximum flow rate occurs in the first quarter of the total voiding time (Fig. 1A). A flow curve, described by a quick rise in flow rate that reaches a peak within 1 s of the initiation of urine flow, is often suggestive of DI.

For the proper interpretation of uroflow parameters, the various factors that can affect urinary flow rate should be considered. For instance, the nonlinear relationship between voided volume and Q_{max} has been well documented (Abrams 1984; Layton and Drach 1983). To manage this problem, nomograms have been developed that enable the comparison of Q_{max} at different voided volumes and can be used to identify abnormal voiding (Siroky et al. 1979). Although Q_{max} is more dependent upon initial bladder volume, this measurement normally requires catheterization to determine postvoid residual volume. Radionuclide techniques have recently been introduced to assess bladder emptying function. The advantage of this method is that both urinary flow rate and residual volume (and thus initial bladder volume) can be determined simultaneously and noninvasively (Groshar et al. 1988, 1991).

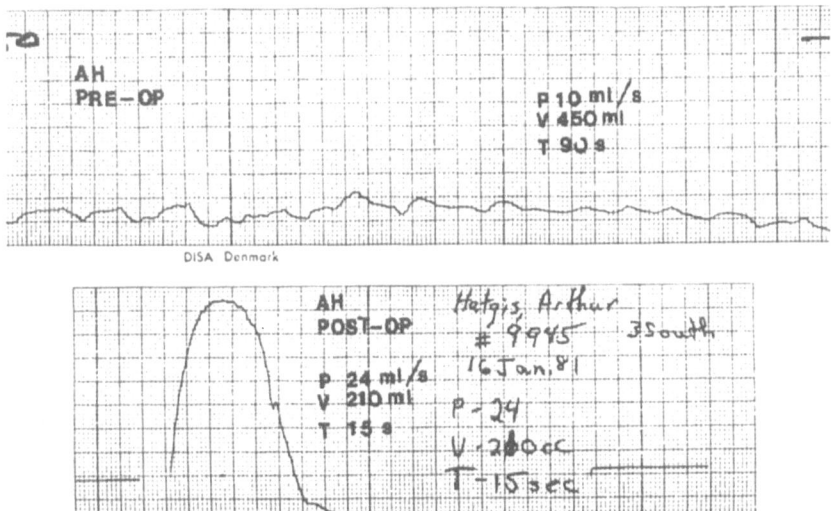

Fig. 1. *Top*: abnormal flow curve from patient with bladder outlet obstruction; Q_{max} = 10 ml/s, voided volume = 450 ml, total voiding time = 90 s. *Bottom*: normal uroflow from same patient after bladder neck incision and prostatotomy. Q_{max} = 24 ml/s, voided volume = 210 ml, voiding time = 15 s

Another factor that influences urinary flow rate is gender (Drach et al. 1979b); Q_{max} in normal women is 5 ml/s higher than that of normal men at a given volume. The effect of age on the voiding parameters remains unresolved. Although studies have shown a 2 ml/s decrease in Q_{max} for every 10 years of age in males (Layton and Drach 1983), this correlation does not hold for aging females. The actual impact of aging on urinary flow rate is difficult to ascertain, given that data from truly normal elderly men are scarce and that other studies find no significant relationship between age and Q_{max} (Drach et al. 1979b). Nomograms are available that, in addition to adjusting for volume voided, also correct for variations in Q_{max} due to age (Drach et al. 1979a) and sex. Additional factors that affect voiding parameters include abdominal straining, which can produce abnormally high Q_{max} and interrupted flow patterns, and psychological inhibition of flow due to anxiety or embarassment induced by the testing environment.

Urinary flow represents the interaction between bladder contraction and outlet resistance to flow. Consequently, flow rates can only be classified as normal or abnormal. Although the presence of outlet obstruction decreases Q_{max}, abnormally low flow rates cannot reliably differentiate between bladder dysfunction (detrusor hypoactivity) and urethral obstruction. Using exclusively Q_{max} as a diagnostic indicator, outlet obstruction can be correctly predicted in only 50% of the cases (Anderson 1982). Therefore, patients with abnormal urinary flows require more sophisticated urodynamic evaluation before effective therapeutic intervention can be initiated. Alternate strategies of therapy (watchful waiting, medical management with α-adrenergic blockade, anticholinergics) can then be recommended for those with severe symptoms of prostatism who are believed to be unobstructed or only minimally obstructed.

Urinary Velocity Measurements

Gleason et al. have advocated the simultaneous measurement of both urinary stream velocity and urinary flow rate as a noninvasive method to more clearly distinguish between normal and obstructed voiding (Gleason et al. 1972; Meyhoff et al. 1989). By directing the urinary stream towards the paddlewheel of a dynamometer, stream velocity can be determined as it is proportional to the speed of paddlewheel rotation (Gleason et al. 1982). These studies have shown that stream velocity, in conjunction with urinary flow, provide a more sensitive method of detecting abnormal urination patterns.

Another method of evaluating the urinary stream, introduced by Zinner et al. , is the urinary drop spectrometer (Zinner et al. 1983). As the urinary stream breaks into a spectrum of drops, each drop is analyzed as it passes between a colli- mated beam of light and the detector. This sophisticated instrument can be used to measure the size and shape of each drop of urine. Measurements of flow rate and drop frequency, which is related to stream velocity, can be obtained from this analysis. These investigators have reported that this technique can discriminate patients with clinical BPH from normal patients based on a single urination in 95% of their cases. Although the drop spectrometer can be used to detect lower urinary tract dysfunction and explore important hydrodynamic properties of urination, the prohibitive costs of the equipment render this method impractical for routine clinical use.

Cystometry

Meaningful information about bladder activity during the filling and storage phases of micturition can be obtained from the cystometrogram. When performed properly, cystometry can reveal the viscoelastic properties, proprioception, capacity, and reflex activity of the bladder. When outlet obstruction is suspected, cystometry is intended, not as a method of determining the presence, location, or magnitude of outlet obstruction, but as a means of assessing the impact of the obstruction on the bladder. Since DI is frequently observed in patients with obstructive BPH, cystometry can provide documentation of the incidence and severity of this disorder. However, the mere confirmation of DI by cystometry is not an acceptable indication for surgical treatment, since DI is also associated with aging (Resnick 1988); thus without urodynamic evidence to the contrary, outlet obstruction cannot be assumed as the underlying cause of DI.

Cystometry requires bladder catheterization, usually with a 10–14F bilumen catheter. The bladder is filled at a predetermined rate through one of the catheter ports while the other is used to measure intravesical pressure via fluid-filled lines connected to a strain gauge transducer. Measurement of intra-abdominal or rectal pressure prevents pressure changes due to abdominal straining, patient movement, or other artifacts from being inadvertently attributed to changes in detrusor compliance or involuntary detrusor contractions. When this study is preceded by uroflowmetry, the postvoid residual volume can easily be measured at the time of catheterization. The patient is made as comfortable as possible and is instructed to vocalize his sensations as the bladder is filled with normal saline (or dilute radiocontrast solution if fluoroscopic facilities are available). The bladder volumes are recorded for each of the following events: first sensation of bladder filling, first sensation of fullness, first desire to void, and urgent desire to void. The resting bladder pressure, the presence and frequency of involuntary detrusor contractions, and pressure at bladder capacity should also be noted. Provocative maneuvers such as coughing, straining, suprapublic tapping, and postural changes can be performed throughout the study to induce involuntary bladder contractions.

During the filling phase, the pressure-volume relationship of the bladder is expressed in terms of its compliance. The normal bladder capacity ranges from 350–500 ml with the first sensation of bladder filling occurring around 150 ml and the first urge to void at 350 ml (Blaivas 1988). Since bladder pressure normally increases by less than 10 cm H_2O at bladder capacity, normal compliance can fall between 35–50 ml/cm H_2O. The typically nonlinear pressure-volume relationship can be accounted for by defining compliance more accurately in terms of bladder volume.

The cystometric curve consists of an initial rise in bladder pressure due to the viscoelastic response to stretch, followed by a relatively stable phase of accommodation to increasing bladder volume. Clinical studies have demonstrated that the shape of the cystometric curve is directly dependent upon the rate of bladder filling (Coolsaet 1985), the bladder viscoelastic properties or the amount of collagen in the bladder wall (Susset et al. 1978), the active properties of the smooth muscle, and the interactions between these factors. A decrease in compliance or an increase in bladder wall stiffness may occur in long-standing obstructions due to collagen deposition and smooth muscle hypertrophy. Similar changes in compliance can occur in detrusor (neurogenic) pathologies or chronic inflammatory processes. These morphological and functional changes may eventually precipitate urinary retention or changes in the upper urinary tract. However, no clinical data are available to support the existence of these potential outcomes.

The evacuation phase of micturition provides the opportunity to examine the quality of the bladder musculature. As the patient initiates voiding, detrusor pressure normally rises to 40–60 cm H_2O and flow begins once the opening pressure is exceeded. Aspects of the contraction to be observed include the voluntary initiation of the contraction, the maximum pressure attained during the contraction, the duration of the contraction, the ability to voluntarily interrupt urination, and augmentation of voiding by abdominal straining. The strength of the detrusor muscle can be objectively assessed by the "stop test" in which either the patient is asked to terminate his stream or a balloon catheter is pulled into the bladder neck. A similar approach, the continuous occlusion test (COT), entails gently occluding the bladder neck prior to the bladder contraction. This technique may eliminate the patient discomfort, inconsistent timing of the occlusion, and possible reflex inhibition associated with the conventional "stop test." From this test, the maximum isometric pressure (P_{iso}) attained during the total occlusion provides an approximation of maximum detrusor strength (Coolsaet and Blok 1986). The maximum velocity of contraction can be calculated from the isometric contraction phase as the fastest change of pressure relative to the detrusor pressure, $(dP/dt)_{max}/P$ (Coolsaet and Blok 1986). Although the clinical significance of these descriptive parameters remains controversial, their role in characterizing the quality of the detrusor contraction and predicting surgical outcome warrants further investigation.

Radiologic and fluoroscopic monitoring during cystometry can add valuable information concerning the functional anatomy of the lower urinary system during urination, particularly regarding the bladder contour (presence of trabeculation, cellules, and diverticula), detrusor contraction, bladder base descent, vesicourethral funnelling, reflux into the prostatic ducts, seminal vesicles and ureters, urethral compliance, bulbous urethral filling and postvoid residual volume (Yalla 1988). The advantages gained by simultaneous pressure monitoring and radiographic visualization of the study profoundly outweigh the additional effort and expense of the technique.

Voiding Cystourethrography

The voiding cystourethrogram (VCUG) is an indispensable diagnostic procedure which can provide valuable information regarding the anatomical and functional features of the lower urinary tract. For urodynamically confirmed outlet obstructions, the VCUG enables the visualization of the precise location of the mechanical constriction. This procedure also permits the functional evaluation of the sphincter mechanism and the identification of detrusor-sphincter dyssynergia. The diagnostic value of the VCUG is dramatically improved when performed in conjunction with cystometry (as discussed previously). Furthermore, the quality and clinical utility of the information extracted from the VCUG depends on the urodynamic experience of the investigator.

The basic hydrodynamic principles of fluid flow through collapsible tube systems provide the basis for understanding the rationale of urodynamic evaluation of the lower urinary tract in general and extracting relevant diagnostic features from the VCUG. In a collapsible tube such as the urethra, the impedance encountered by the contracting bladder is determined by a segment of the urethra known as the flow-controlling zone which uncouples the bladder and the distal urethra (Griffiths 1988). The funnel configuration of the proximal urethra gives rise to the narrowing of the flow-controlling zone, causing energy dissipation and a drop in hydrostatic pressure. In the area of the flow-controlling zone, fluid velocity is sonic (relative to the velocity of elastic waves of the urethra). The transition from subsonic to supersonic flow velocity in this constricted region is followed by a distention of the urethra that is associated with local turbulence. The return to subsonic flow – the elastic jump – may occur here, near the distal end of the membranous urethra (Yalla et al. 1985). Urinary flow is independent of the properties of the distal urethra since transmission of downstream disturbances are prevented by the proximal flow-controlling zone. In general, the flow rate depends on the detrusor pressure, the elastic properties of the flow-controlling zone, and the energy loss across the prostatic urethra (Griffiths 1971).

In normal adults, the bladder contour appears smooth, with a well-funneled bladder neck and prostatic fossa, a well-filled bulbous urethra, and no evidence of the elastic jump (Fig. 2). In patients with hypocontractile detrusor function or habitual Valsalva voiders, radiographic evidence typically indicates large capacity bladders that descend into the pelvis with incomplete relaxation of the external sphincter; angulation or kinking at the prostatomembranous junction is sometimes observed in those with prolonged conditions. Often, reflux into the prostatic ducts (Fig. 3) with incomplete filling of the bulbous urethra can be detected on these films. In patients with chronic calculous prostatitis, reflux, and the associated prostatic calculi and incomplete relaxation or spasm of the external sphincter are observed. Severe outlet obstruction can be radiologically characterized by heavily trabeculated bladders (frequently with diverticulum formation), underfilling of the proximal bulbous urethra and inadequate funneling of the bladder neck as shown in Fig. 4. After the patient voids, preferably in privacy, a postvoid film will demonstrate the efficiency of bladder emptying. Evidence of the elastic jump at the

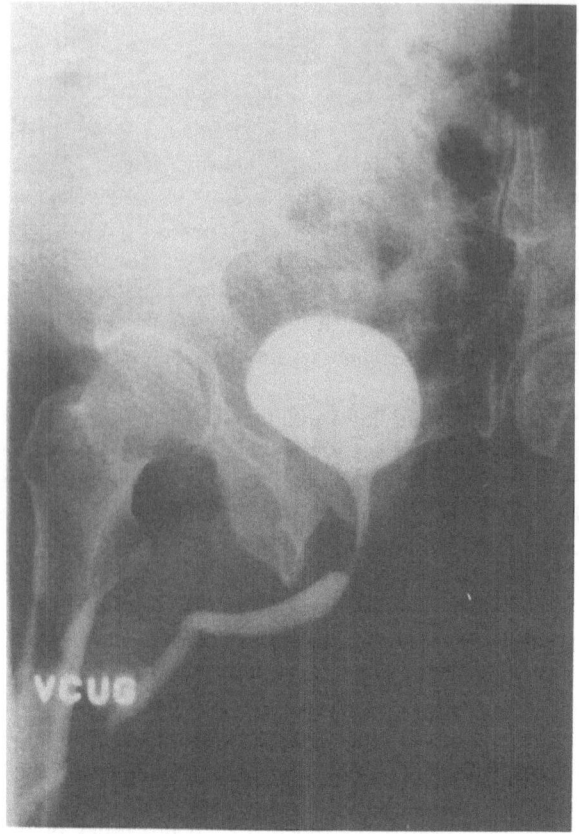

Fig. 2. Normal voiding cystourethography (VCUG) illustrating smooth contoured bladder, a well funneled bladder neck, and a distended bulbous urethra

proximal bulbous urethra which appears narrow and inadequately filled can be seen in severe prostatic or bladder neck obstructions or severe membranous urethral obstructions secondary to the striated sphincter spasticity of dyssynergia (Fig. 5). This elastic jump, with underfilling of the proximal bulb, can be eliminated by additional distal urethral constrictions.

By observing the entire voiding process under fluoroscopic control, from initiation of micturition to the point of its cessation, conditions such as detrusor-sphincter dyssynergia and Valsalva voiding due to hyporeflexic detrusor dysfunction can often be recognized. Although the VCUG offers some indications about the anatomical and functional characteristics of the lower urinary tract, it may not provide a complete understanding of the nature of the voiding dysfunction. For example, the VCUG from a patient with a hypocontractile bladder may demonstrate poor opacification of the prostatic urethra, inadequate funneling of the bladder neck, and inadequate filling of the bulbous urethra, but it cannot rule out a coexisting

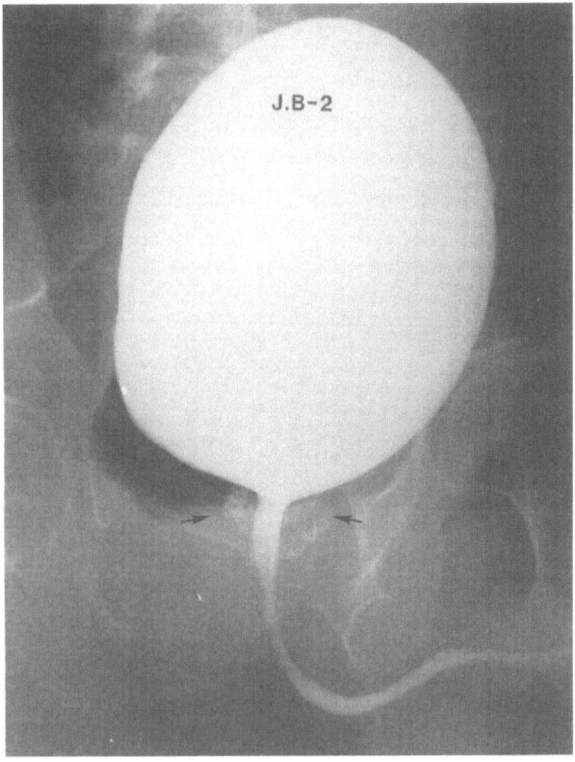

Fig. 3. Voiding cystourethography (VCUG) of patient with large capacity, hypocontractile bladder who voids with Valsalva. Prostatic reflux is shown with *two arrows*. The bulb is inadequately filled, suggesting partial relaxation of striated sphincter

outlet obstruction in the posterior urethra or differentiate a poorly contracting bladder from a mild outlet obstruction. Under these circumstances, further urodynamic studies are essential to accurately characterize the nature of the voiding dysfunction.

Voiding Profilometry

For patients with prostatism symptoms and equivocal uroflow findings, voiding profilometry is an integral component of advanced urodynamic evaluation. This procedure is particularly useful in determining the location, severity, and type of outlet compromise and can be instrumental in eliminating obstruction as a cause of symptoms in patients with severe DI and low volume-low flow urinations (Yalla 1983).

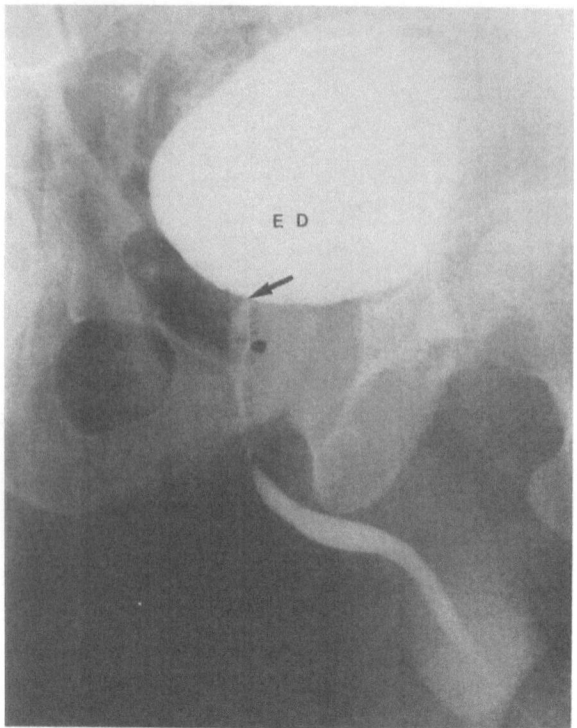

Fig. 4. Voiding cystourethography (VCUG) of patient with prostatic obstruction showing a narrow, irregular prostatic urethra (*arrow*) and poor filling of the bulbous urethra

The primary concept of voiding profilometry or the micturitional vesico-urethral pressure profile (MUPP) is to record hydrostatic pressure along the entire lower urinary tract during established urination (Yalla et al. 1980). By means of a 10F triple lumen catheter, simultaneous intravesical pressure and the hydrostatic pressure of the lower bladder segment, the bladder neck, the prostatic, membranous, and bulbous and penile urethra are recorded, preferably under fluoroscopic control. The two channels which terminate separately at the catheter tip are used for bladder filling and pressure recording, while the third channel, terminating in two side-hole ports located 10–15 cm from the catheter tip, is used to monitor urethral pressure via the Brown and Wickham infusion principle (Brown and Wickham 1969). Radiopaque markers located at the tip of the catheter and at the site of the urethral port facilitate the identification of functional and anatomical landmarks in relation to the calibrated marks on the catheter during urethral pressure profilometry. As the catheter is slowly withdrawn in centimeter increments under resting bladder conditions, the bladder neck and external sphincter can be identified as the first rise in pressure and the maximum pressure, respectively, in the urethral closure pressure profile.

The catheter is reintroduced fully into the bladder and filling is continued until the patient senses a strong urge to void. During the mid-voiding phase, the catheter is again withdrawn gently at 0.5 cm/s so that pressures are recorded simultaneously in the bladder and along the part of the urethra of interest (Fig. 6). The accuracy of this analysis requires the continuous monitoring of intravesical pressure to ensure that a urethral pressure drop is effected by the urethral constriction and not by a decrease in detrusor pressure. In normal males, voiding profilometry displays essentially isobaric pressures between the bladder, vesicourethral junction, and proximal prostatic urethra as shown in Fig. 7. A physiologic drop in pressure occurs near the apex of the prostate and the narrow membranous urethra which functions as the flow-controlling zone. (In elastic tubes, such as the urethra, the maximum flow rate is limited by the elastic properties of this narrow compressive zone in which the speed of the fluid reaches sonic velocity (Griffiths 1971).)

The MUPP obtained from an obstructed patient is certainly distinct from that of the normal patient (Fig. 8). The shape of the pressure profile depends on the anatomical distribution of the prostatic enlargement along the posterior urethra and the extent of the mechanical obstruction. The location of the obstruction can be identified at the drop in hydrostatic pressure at a site in the prostatic urethra that depends upon the location of the most constrictive segment of the prostatic enlargement. This apparent pressure drop is predominantly due to an increase in upstream (detrusor) pressure unless detrusor contractility is abnormal. The severity of the prostatic obstruction then determines the site of the flow-controlling zone. In cases of mild to moderate obstruction, profilometry will reveal a second drop in pressure in the vicinity of the external sphincter or the urogenital diaphragm which remains the flow-controlling zone. However, severe prostatic obstructions will reestablish the flow-controlling zone proximally, thus concealing the second drop at the external sphincter. Similarly, if the constriction appears in the penile urethra, depending on the severity of the constriction, the drop in pressure across the membranous urethra will be obscured by the pressure change across the relocated flow-controlling zone in the penile urethra. When attempting to evaluate the magnitude of the pressure change across a constriction, both the severity of the constriction and the bladder contractile performance should be considered.

An index of relative obstruction has been proposed which includes the contributions of detrusor contractility performance and the outlet conduit properties (Sullivan et al. 1992). The detrusor contractility is represented by the peak detrusor pressure generated (P_{iso}) with complete outlet occlusion (COT). This is accomplished with a 10F balloon catheter with the balloon inflated and secured in the bladder neck. The relative obstruction index (ROI) is calculated from the following formula: ROI = MUPP/P_{iso}, where MUPP is the pressure drop across the bladder neck and the prostatic urethra and P_{iso} is the maximum isometric detrusor pressure reached during bladder occlusion. As an example, a minor degree of outlet compression or constriction (small pressure drop on MUPP) can be expressed as a severe degree of relative obstruction (high ROI) if accompanied by poor detrusor

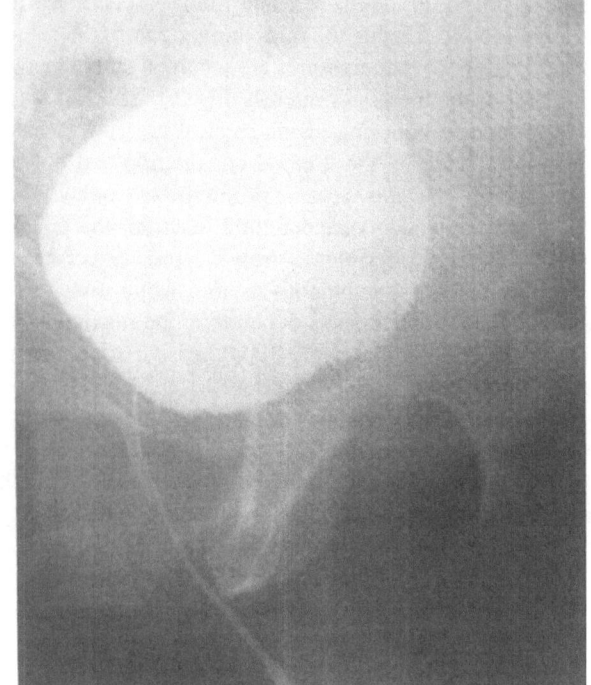

A

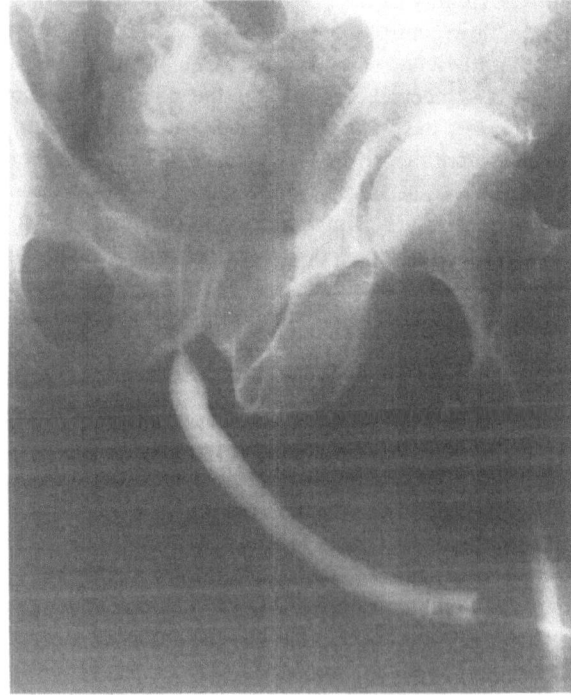

B

Fig. 5A and B

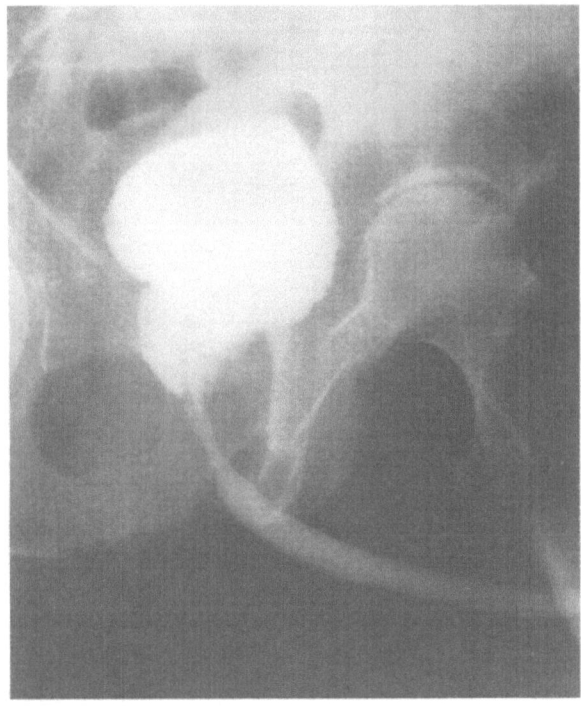

C

Fig. 5. A Voiding cystourethography (VCUG) of patient with urodynamically confirmed severe prostatic obstruction. Note collapse, nondistended bulbous urethra, and long elastic jump. **B** Retrograde urethrogram of patient same patient illustrating the anatomical position of proximal bulb and its distensibility. **C** Postoperative VCUG of same patient which shows extensive resection of the prostatic urethra, complete filling of the proximal bulb, and proximal migration of elastic jump

contraction pressure (P_{iso}). However, this same pressure drop may not be significant if the detrusor has normal contractility, in which case the ROI will be correspondingly smaller. This single quantitative parameter can characterize the relative severity of functional impairment and may provide a useful method of assessing treatment outcomes by measuring changes in the ROI.

The effect of catheter size on the pressure measurement should be considered in the analysis of pressure profilometry and has therefore been investigated experimentally (Yalla et al. 1981a). No statistical difference was found between pressure profiles obtained with a 5F or a 10F catheter in normal subjects. However, catheter size may become critical in severe cases of prostatic obstruction in which upstream pressures may become further exaggerated by catheter compromise. Since the use of a 5F catheter would preclude the simultaneous measurement of bladder pressure or would require insertion of a suprapubic cannula, the advantages of a larger triple lumen catheter (10F) far exceed its drawbacks in most cases.

Previous experimental studies have confirmed that MUPP is a reliable and dependable technique that enables the documentation of abnormal urethral constrictions or compression sites in the urethra (Yalla and Resnick 1984; Yalla et al.

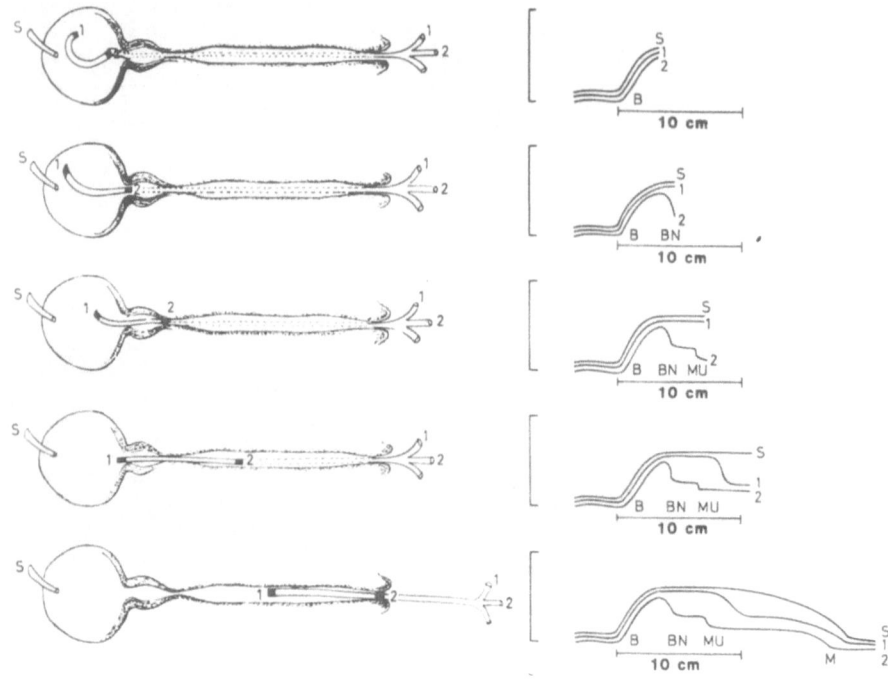

Rate of pull 1cm/2-5s

Fig. 6. Catheter withdrawal technique and respective pressure configurations during micturition in a patient with a bladder neck obstruction. *S*, suprapubic cannula; *B*, bladder; *BN*, bladder neck; *MU*, membranous urethra; *M*, meatus. Static pressure drop is recorded at the *BN* and *MU* through two lateral ports (*1, 2*) of the catheter

1980). This method is especially advantageous for patients in which the use of advanced urodynamics is impractical or technically cumbersome, particularly the frail elderly and those with spinal cord injury or limited mobility (Sotolongo and Nelson 1990). However, the MUPP cannot be applied in patients who have an areflexic or acontractile detrusor since the passive properties of the outlet cannot be assessed without a detrusor contraction, striated sphincter relaxation, and urinary flow. The MUPP continues to be used clinically to assess vesical outlet dysfunctions resulting from isolated bladder neck (Yalla et al. 1981b), benign prostatic enlargements (Yalla et al. 1981c), detrusor-sphincter dyssynergia (Yalla et al. 1982), and anterior urethral strictures (Yalla and Loughlin 1982). Methods have also been introduced to determine the severity of the obstruction based on the calculated diameter and resistance of the presumed "near rigid" segment of the constricted urethra (Asklin et al. 1984). In addition, a good correlation has been reported between the MUPP and standard pressure-flow studies for diagnosing outlet obstruction (Desmond and Ramayya 1988).

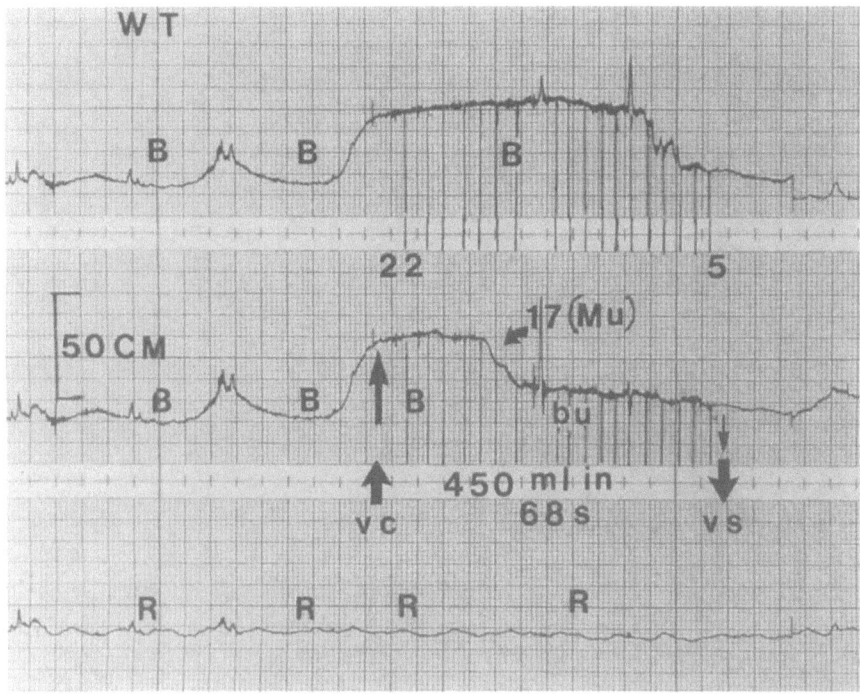

Fig. 7. Micturitional vesicourethral pressure profile (MUPP) from patient with a virtually normal configuration. *Top panel*: continous recording of bladder pressure during micturition; *vertical lines* represent
1 cm of catheter withdrawal; *Middle panel*: vesicourethral static pressure profile showing roughly
isobaric bladder (*B*) and urethral pressures until physiologic pressure drop across membranous urethra
(*Mu*); *VC*, voiding commences; *bu*, bulbous urethra; *vs*, voiding stops. *Bottom panel*: rectal (*R*) pressure

Endourodynamics

Attempts to improve traditional urodynamic methods, as well as advances in optics
technology, have led to the introduction of endoscopy-aided urodynamic procedures
(Loughlin and Yalla 1986). For these sophisticated studies, a custom-made, 10.5F
flexible fiberoptic endoscope with 5 cm calibration marks on the surface (Olympus
Corporation, New Hyde Park, NY) was introduced into the urethra under local
anesthesia. The endoscope consisted of three channels, each terminating at the tip
of the instrument; two of the channels were reserved for the necessary optics and
illumination while the third was utilized for monitoring total urethral pressure and
fluid infusion.

Although this method is not without its faults, endourodynamics does provide
an interesting addition to the urodynamic armamentarium and offers several

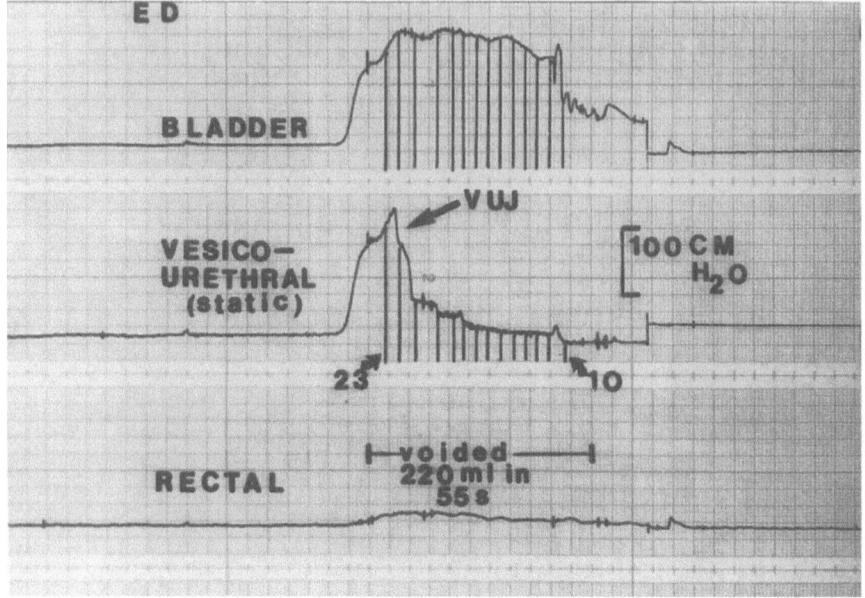

Fig. 8. Micturitional vesicourethral pressure profile (MUPP) of elderly man with severe symptoms of prostatism. *Top panel*: bladder pressure during micturition. *Middle panel*: vesicourethral static pressure profile which shows large pressure drop at vesicourethral junction (*VUJ*) and slight drop at external sphincter zone. *Bottom panel*: rectal pressure

advantages over traditional methods. For instance, the intraurethral anatomy can be visualized endoscopically while urethral pressure is measured during micturition. In addition, radiologic exposure during the urodynamic study can be eliminated and accurate functional evaluations of the bladder outlet can be performed under direct vision through the voiding pressure profile and voiding cystoscopy.

Pressure-Flow Analysis

Indications for more advanced urodynamics procedures such as pressure-flow studies include the assessment of detrusor dysfunctions and the precise diagnosis and evaluation of the severity of outlet obstruction when routine urodynamic studies fail to provide sufficient information. In normal patients, normal flow rates are achieved with lower detrusor pressures. However, increased detrusor pressures associated with decreased flow rates are often observed in patients with outlet obstruction. In certain patients in which the detrusor pressure and the flow rates are both abnormally low, simple cystometry and uroflowmetry cannot provide an accurate differentiation between a hypocontractile bladder, outlet obstruction, and a combination of both pathologies. Although pressure-flow ($P - Q$) studies can be used to identify an obstructed system or define detrusor contractile function, these studies do not provide the location of the obstruction site. Simultaneous fluoroscopic monitoring of the study can, however, assist in confirming the location of the obstruction.

Initial attempts to describe the relationship between pressure and flow resulted in the formulation of resistance (R) coefficients ($R = P_{\text{ves}}/Q$ or $R = P_{\text{ves}}/Q^2$). Since these equations are based on the assumptions that the bladder is perfectly spherical and the urethra functions as a rigid tube, objections concerning the use of these resistance factors have been raised repeatedly (Schäfer 1985, 1986). These investigators have advocated replacing the misused term "urethral resistance" with more rigorous terms that will faithfully describe the flow-determining properties of the urethra.

Various analyses of $P - Q$ studies have been introduced, which depend extensively on the simultaneous, accurate measurement of bladder pressure and urinary flow (Fig. 9). These variables are represented graphically as pressure vs flow after correcting for the time delay inherent in flow measuring devices. The interpretation of data obtained from $P - Q$ studies is based on hydrodynamic principles of flow through elastic tubes in which urethral properties are determined primarily by the distensibility of the flow-controlling zone in the urethra. To analyze $P - Q$ studies, explicit hydrodynamic concepts have been introduced to separate the contributions of the bladder from that of the urethra, consequently enabling the evaluation of outlet obstruction independent from detrusor contraction strength.

Schäfer's analysis of $P - Q$ data provides a quantitative description of bladder outlet function due to the morphologic tissue properties – the passive urethral resistance relation (PURR) – and dynamic changes in the outlet caused by muscular contraction or relaxation during micturition, the dynamic urethral resistance relation (DURR). The PURR is a curve described by the polynomial regression of the borderline of lowest resistance on the $P - Q$ plot (Fig. 10). Deviations from these optimal outflow conditions are represented as a function of time in the DURR plot (Schäfer 1983).

Relevant to the interpretation of this model is the concept of the minimum urethral opening pressure (P_{muo}). In the passive state, the urethra is completely collapsed with the coapted surfaces of the soft mucosal lining giving the urethral lumen its distinctive configuration and creating a sealing effect (Zinner et al. 1980). The urethral elasticity and its intraluminal pressure govern the effective cross-sectional area of the lumen. Therefore, during the initiation of micturition when the urethra is completely relaxed, bladder pressure must attain the minimum intraurethral fluid pressure required to open and maintain the urethral lumen before fluid can enter the proximal urethra. This minimum urethral opening pressure (P_{muo}), which can be easily determined from the P vs Q plot, is an estimation of the pressure at the flow-controlling zone during the initiation of flow and, for the perfectly elastic urethra, at the termination of flow. Consequently, a fraction of the available bladder pressure is required at the flow-controlling zone to keep the urethral lumen open and thus cannot be converted into fluid flow velocity.

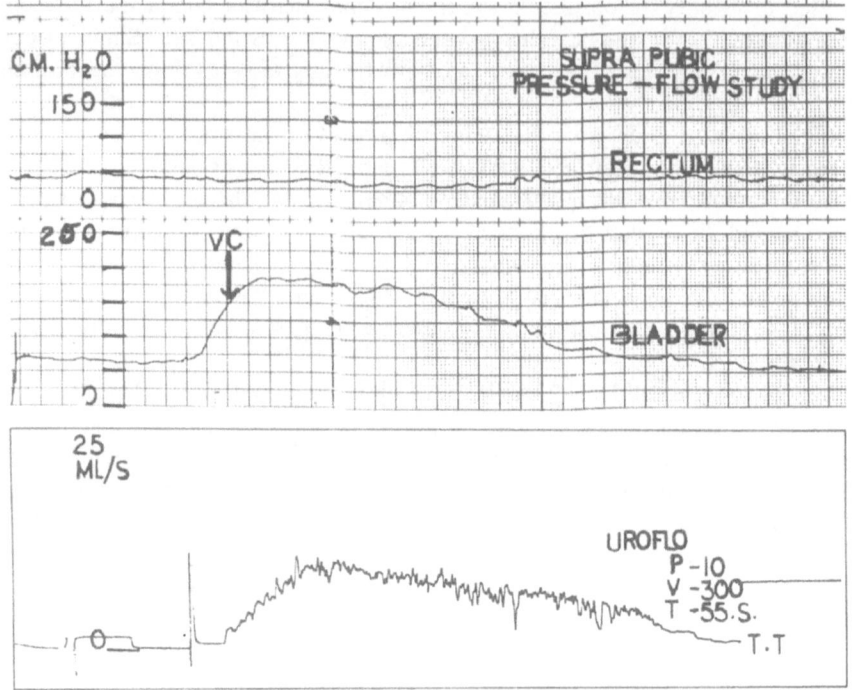

Fig. 9. Synchronous pressure-flow study. *Top panel*: rectal pressure. *Middle panel*: bladder pressure measured with suprapubic cannula. *Bottom panel*: uroflow; $Q_{max} = 10$ ml/s, voided volume = 300 ml, total voiding time = 55 S. This patient had high detrusor pressure and low flow rate, suggesting bladder outlet obstruction. Micturitional vesicourethral pressure profile (MUPP) has shown isolated bladder neck obstruction which was treated with incision

In this model, the distended lumen in the flow-controlling urethra is regarded as a tube with constant static pressure and constant cross-sectional area. The $P - Q$ relation during urination under optimal outflow conditions can be effectively described by the relative slope (c) and intercept (P_{muo}) of the PURR curve defined as $P_{det} = P_{muo} + c^{-1}Q^2$ (Schäfer 1983). From the Bernoulli equation and the continuity equation, the value obtained for c can be used to calculate the effective cross-sectional area of the flow-controlling zone: $CA = (c\rho/2)^{1/2}$, where CA is the cross-sectional area and ρ is the density of the fluid.

Griffiths has reduced the $P - Q$ data to a single group specific urethral resistance factor (URA) to quantify urethral function during micturition (Griffiths et al. 1989). This one-parameter model is empirically derived from the positive correlation that was found between the P_{muo} and the slope of the $P - Q$ curve, thus integrating these parameters into one descriptive term. Within a particular group of patients with a specific type of obstruction, this value of URA at peak flow can be used to quantitatively compare and grade the degree of "urethral resistance."

A more complex model of the relationship between detrusor pressure and urinary flow or area of the flow-controlling zone has been developed by Spanberg et al.

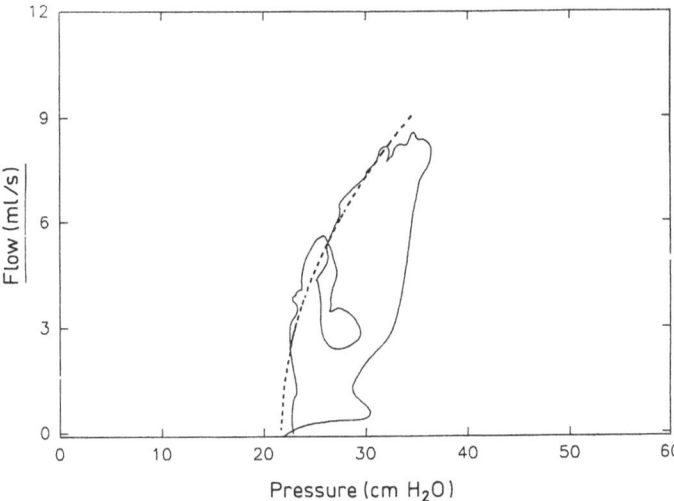

Fig. 10. Plot of detrusor pressure vs flow during micturition. The passive urethral resistance relation is superimposed with *dotted line*

(1989). In this model, urethral function can be fully characterized by the urethral opening pressure, urethral lumen cross-sectional area and urethral elasticity. Three descriptive parameters from the following equation, $P_{det} = P_{muo} + L_m Q_m$, the opening pressure ($P_{muo}$), slope ($L_m$), and shape ($m$) of the curve, are estimated analytically from a least squares method of curves fitting the $P - Q$ plot. This analysis can establish the severity of an obstruction and can also be used to identify the biomechanical changes that may be associated with obstruction, thus distinguishing constrictive and compressive obstructions (Fig. 11) and describing the compliant properties of the obstructed site. Obstructive conditions characterized by an elevated P_{muo} imply that a larger fraction of the total available bladder energy is required to maintain a distended flow-controlling zone. Once opened, the urethra has normal compliance in this "compressive" type of obstruction. In "low-compliant" obstructions, an elevated L_m is coupled with a low m, such that a higher static pressure (above the P_{muo}) is needed to expand the flow-controlling zone. A "constrictive" type of obstruction, in which both L_m and m are elevated, is associated with a normally distended urethra which requires a significant increase in pressure for further expansion. Preoperative evaluation of BPH patients in this study classified most of the urethral dysfunctions as compressive obstructions combined with either low-compliant or constrictive components (Spangberg et al. 1991). Postoperative studies of these patients revealed a reduction in P_{muo} and slope of the $P - Q$ relation; however, the curve retained its low-compliant or constrictive shape, suggesting that the distensibility of the flow-controlling zone is restricted by fibrosis at the distal resection margin.

The results of $P - Q$ studies cannot account for all prostatism symptoms or predict whether these symptoms will be alleviated by surgical intervention.

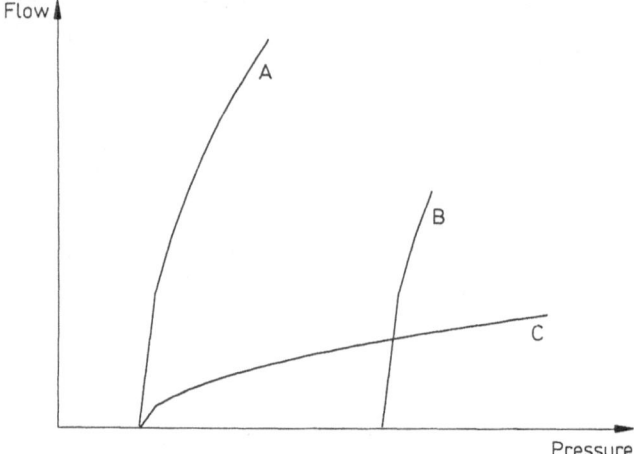

Fig. 11. Passive urethral resistance relation for different types of constrictions. *A*, Normal passive urethral resistance relation (PURR); *B*, compressive obstruction; *C*, constrictive obstruction

Simultaneous $P - Q$ studies by Abrams et al. (1981) showed that symptomatic improvement occurred in about 88% of the patients treated with TURP compared with 72% improvement in a group of postoperative patients who were not evaluated by $P - Q$ studies. Jansen's analysis of $P - Q$ studies has shown symptomatic improvement in 93% of obstructed patients, whereas, 78% of unobstructed men show substantial improvement following TURP (Jensen et al. 1988). Their study did not show any difference in mean symptom scores between the obstructed and the unobstructed patients after surgery. Analysis of $P - Q$ studies by Schäfer et al. (1989) has shown a significant postprostatectomy improvement in flow rate and residual volume only in patients with objective evidence of severe obstruction. Other studies have shown that men with low flow rates and high voiding pressures (greater than 80 cm H_2O) were more likely to have a good subjective outcome than patients with lower voiding pressures and low flow rates (Neal et al. 1989). Although many of these studies suggest that men who are objectively obstructed as determined by $P - Q$ analysis, have better outcomes following surgery, the question of who should benefit from surgical intervention is only confounded by the documentation of at least some postoperative improvement in unobstructed men. The precise mechanisms responsible for postoperative alleviation of symptoms in patients with nonobstructive prostates remain obscure.

These $P - Q$ analyses have contributed greatly to the effort of establishing better indications for surgical treatment of prostatism and developing improved correlations between urodynamic data and symptomatology. Computer software designed to analyze these pressure and flow signals has recently been incorporated into commercially available urodynamic equipment. Clinically relevant urodynamic parameters can be automatically obtained with these programs and directly used for patient management. However, some of the practical limitations of this methodology are disturbing. These studies are somewhat invasive and require the cooperation of the patient, experienced personnel, and specialized urodynamic instrumentation. Therefore, interpretable data are often very difficult to obtain, even by skilled researchers. Although advances in technology and improvements in urodynamic equipment will alleviate some of these problems, further studies are necessary to ascertain the clinical utility of these advanced methods.

With our understanding of hydrodynamic principles and given the currently available urodynamic techniques, we initially screen our patients with prostatism with a good clinical history, a thorough neurological evaluation, uroflowmetry, and a fluoroscopically monitored VCUG. By employing these techniques, we are able to detect, in the majority of our patients, clear-cut abnormalities of vesicourethral dysfunction (obstructive and non-obstructive). Patients with normal flow rates and minimal morphologic and functional disturbances are treated conservatively and followed. Abnormal detrusor function and ambiguous outlet obstructions demonstrated with VCUG are studied further with voiding profilometry and/or $P - Q$ studies. This approach enables the judicious treatment of all of our patients with prostatism.

References

Abrams PH, Farrar DJ, Turner-Warwick RT et al. (1981) The results of prostatectomy: a symptomatic and urodynamic analysis of 152 patients. J Urol 125:640–642

Abrams P (1984) The practice of urodynamics. In: Mundy, AR, Stephenson, TP, Wein, AJ (eds) Urodynamics. Principles, practice and application. Churchill Livingstone, New York, pp 76–92

Anderson JT (1982) Prostatism: clinical, radiological, and urodynamic aspects. Neurourol Urodyn 1:241–293

Asklin B, Erlandson BE, Johansson G, Pettersson S (1984) The Micturitional Urethral Pressure Profile. Scand J Urol Nephrol. 18:269–276

Blaivas JG (1988) Techniques of evaluation. In: Yalla, SV, McGuire, EJ, Elbadawi, A, Blaivas, JG (eds) Neurourology and urodynamics. Macmillan, New York, pp 155–198

Brown M, Wickham JEA (1969) The urethral pressure profile. Br J Urol 41:211–217

Coolsaet, B (1985) Bladder compliance and detrusor activity during the collection phase. Neurourol Urodyn 4:263–274

Coolsaet B, Block C (1986) Detrusor Properties Related to Prostatism. Neurourol Urodyn 5:435–447

Cucchi A (1988) Detrusor instability and bladder outflow obstruction: evidence for a correlation between the severity of obstruction and the presence of instability. Br J Urol 61:420–422

Desmond AD, Ramayya GR (1988) Comparison of pressure/flow studies with micturitional urethral pressure profiles in the diagnosis of urinary ourflow obstruction. Br J Urol 61:224–229

Drach GW, Layton TN, Binard WJ (1979a) Male Peak Urinary Flow Rate: Relationships to Volume and Age. J Urol 122:210–214

Drach GW, Ingnatoff J, Layton P (1979b) Peak urinary flow rate: observations in female subjects and comparison to male subjects. J Urol 122:215–219

Dyro, FM, DuBeau, CE, Sullivan, MP, Cravalho, EG, Yalla, SV (1992) Covert co-morbid neurologic abnormalities in patients with symptoms of prostatism. J Urol (in press)

Gleason, DM, Bottaccini, MR, Reilly, RJ, Byrne, JC (1972) The residual stream energy is a diagnostic index of male urinary outflow obstruction. Invest Urol 10:72–77

Gleason, DM, Bottaccini, MR, Drach, GW, Layton, TN (1982) Urinary flow velocity as and index of male voiding function. J Urol 128:1363–1367

Griffiths, DJ (1971) Hydrodynamics of male micturition - I. Theory of steady flow through elastic-walled tubes. Med. Biol. Eng 9:581–588

Griffiths, DG (1988) Mechanics of micturition. In: Yalla, SV, McGuire, EJ, Elbadawi, A, Blaivas, JG (eds) Neurourology and urodynamics. Macmillan, New York, pp 96–105

Griffiths, D, van Mastrigt, R, Bosch, R (1989) Quantification of urethral resistance and bladder function during voiding, with special reference to the effects of prostate size reduction on urethral obstruction due to benign prostatic hyperplasia. Neurourol Urodyn 8:17-27

Groshar, D, Embon, OM, Sazbon, A, Koritny, ES, Frenkel, A (1988) Radionuclide assessment of bladder outlet obstruction: a noninvasive (1-step) method for measurement of voiding time, urinary flow rates and residual urine. J Urol 139:266-269

Groshar, D, Sazbon, Al, Embon, OM, Frenkel, A, Koritny, ES (1991) Radionuclide assessment of bladder-emptying function in normal male population and in patients before and after prostatectomy. Urodynamics 37:353-357

Jensen, K, Bruskewitz, RC, Iversen, P, et al. (1983) Significance of prostatic weight in prostatism. Urol Int. 38:173-178

Jensen, K M-E, Morgensen, JB, Morgensen, P (1988) Urodynamics in prostatism II: prognostic values of pressure-flow study combined with stop-flow test. Scand. J Urol Nephrol. [Suppl] 114:72-77

Jensen, K M-E, Jorgensen, JB, Morgensen P (1988) Urodynamics in prostatism III: prognostic value of medium-fill cystometry. Scand. J Urol Nephrol. [Suppl] 114:78-83

Klarskov, P, Anderson, JT, Asmussen, CF, et al. (1987) Symptoms and signs predictive of voiding pattern after acute urinary retention. Scand. J Urol Nephrol. 21:23-28

Layton, TN, Drach, G (1983) Urinary Flow Rates. In:Hinman, F (ed) Benign prostatic hypertrophy. Springer, Berlin Heidelberg New York, pp 523-527

Lepor, H, Gilbert, R (1990) The efficacy of transurethral resection of the prostate in men with moderate symptoms of prostatism. J Urol 143:533-537

Loughlin, KR, Yalla, SV (1986) Endourodynamics: another valuable dimension in clinical urodynamics. Neurourol Urodyn 5:291-297

Meyhoff, H-H, Gleason, DM, Bottaccini, MR (1989) The effects of transurethral resection on the urodynamic of prostatism. J Urol 142:785-789

Neal, DE, Ramsden, PD, Sharples, L, et al. (1989) Outcome of elective prostatectomy. Br Med J 299:762-767

Resnick, NM (1988) Voiding dysfunction in the elderly. In: Yalla, SV, McGuire, EJ, Elbadawi, A, et al. (eds) Neurourology and urodynamics: principles and practice. Macmillan, New York, pp 303-330

Schäfer, W (1983) The contribution of the bladder outlet to the relation between pressure and flow rate during micturition. In:Hinman, F Jr (ed) Benign Prostatic Hypertrophy. Springer, Berlin Heidelberg New York, pp 470-496

Schäfer, W (1985) Urethral resistance? Urodynamic concepts of physiological and pathological bladder outlet function during voiding. Neurourol Urodyn 4:161-201

Schäfer, W (1986) Urethral resistance - a misleading term. Neurourol Urodyn 5:271-272

Schäfer, W, Noppeney, R, Rubben, H, Lutzeyer, W (1988) The value of free flow rate and pressure/flow-studies in the routine investigation of BPH patients. Neurourol Urodyn 7:219-221

Schäfer, W, Rubben, H, Noppeney, R, et al. (1989) Obstructed and unobstructed prostatic obstruction: a plea for urodynamic objectivation of bladder outflow obstruction in Benign Prostatic Hyperplasia. World J Urol 6:198-203

. Siroky, MB, Olsson, CA, Krane, RJ (1979) Flow rate nomogram. 1. Development. J Urol 122:665-668

Sotolongo, JR, Nelson, S (1990) The micturitional urethral pressure profile in the diagnosis of obstruction in patients with neurogenic bladder. Neurourol Urodyn 9:211

Spangberg, A, Terio, H, Engberg, A, Ask, P (1989) Quantification of urethral function based on Griffiths' model of flow through elastic tubes. Neurourol Urodyn 8:29-52

Spangberg, A, Terio, H, Ask, P, Engberg, A (1991) Pressure/flow studies preoperatively and postoperatively in patients with Benign Prostatic Hypertrophy: estimation of the urethral pressure/flow relation and urethral elasticity. Neurourol Urodyn 10:139-167

Sullivan, MP, Yalla, SV, DuBeau, CE, Venegas, JG, Cravalho, EG (1992) Obstruction indices derived from micturitional urethral pressure profile (MUPP) and maximal detrusor contraction. AUA meeting 1992; Washington, DC. J Urol p 269, abstract # 222

Susset, JG, Servot-Viguier, D, Lany, F, Madernas, P, Black, R (1978) Collagen in 155 human bladders. Invest Urol 16:204-206

Turner-Warwick, R, Whiteside, CG, Arnold, EP, Bates, EP, Worth, PHL, Milroy, EJG, Webster, JR, Weir, J (1973) A urodynamic view of prostatic obstruction and the results of prostatectomy. Br J Urol 45:631-645

Yalla, SV, (1983) Urethral static pressure profile. In: Hinman F, JR (ed) Benign prostatic hypertrophy, Chapt 56. Springer-Verlag, New York Berlin Heidelberg, pp 577-588

Yalla, SV, (1988) Clinical evaluation of outlet obstruction. In:Yalla, SV, McGuire, EJ, Elbadawi, A, Blaivas, JG (eds) Neurourology and urodynamics. Macmillan, New York, pp 199-210

Yalla, SV, Loughlin, KR (1982) Urodynamic assessment of anterior urethral constrictions. Urology 19:106–113

Yalla, SV, Resnick, NM (1984) Vesicourethral static pressure profile during voiding: methodology and clinical utility. World J Urol 2:196–202

Yalla, SV, Sharma, GVRK, Barsamian, EM (1980) Micturitional static urethral pressure profile: a method of recording urethral pressure profile during voiding and the implication. J Urol 124:649–656

Yalla, SV, Blute, RD, Snyder, H, Yap, W, Fraser, L, Friedman, E (1981a) Isolated bladder neck obstruction of undetermined etiology (primary) in adult male. Urology 17:99–108

Yalla, SV, Waters, WB, Snyder, H, Varady, S, Blute, R (1981b) Urodynamic localization of isolated bladder neck obstruction in men: studies with micturitional vesicourethral static pressure profiles. J Urol 125:677–684

Yalla, SV, Blute, R, Waters, WB, Snyder, H, Fraser, L (1981c) Urodynamic evaluation of prostatic enlargements with micturitional vesicourethral static pressure profiles. J Urol 125:685–689

Yalla, SV, Yap, W, Fam, BA (1982) Detrusor urethral sphincter dyssynergia: micturitional vesicourethral pressure profile patterns. J Urol 128:969–973

Yalla, SV, Cravalho, E, Resnick, N, Chiang, R, Gilliam, J, Brown, K (1985) Elastic jump in male urethra during voiding: clinical observations in male subjects and experimental studies in dogs. J Urol 134:907–913

Zinner, R, Sterling, AM, Ritter, RC (1980) Urology 16:115–117

Zinner, NR, Sterling, AM, Ritter, RC (1983) The urinary drop spectrometer in diagnosis. In:Hinman, F Jr (ed) Benign Prostatic Hypertrophy. Springer, Berlin Heidelberg New York, pp 553–558

Transurethral Incision of the Prostate

M.Riehmann and R.Bruskewitz

Historical Background

Transurethral surgery of the prostate and bladder neck is an old procedure for the treatment of infravesical obstruction. Paré, in 1575, used a metal sound when performing transurethral surgery for infravesical obstruction (Shelley 1969). Through a perineal urethrotomy, Blizzard, in 1806, introduced incision of the prostate using a double gorget or knife (Blain 1983). Guthrie, Bell, Civiale, and Mercier all were strong advocates of transurethral surgery to relieve bladder outlet obstruction and each constructed an instrument of his own. The instruments were called by various names such as prostatome, incisor, excisor, prostatolithotrite, and kiotome. In spite of the refinement of this blind transurethral prostatic surgery at that time, this procedure never became widely accepted, primarily due to the high incidence of infection, bleeding, incontinence, and operative mortality.

Progress in endoscopic prostatic surgery was not accomplished before three major discoveries were made. Edison's development of the lamp in 1879, Hertz' discovery of high frequency current in 1888, and construction of endoscopic instruments, such as the punch by Young in 1909 (Young 1913). Bumpus, in 1926, cut a fenestrum in the cystoscope sheath, and finally, the same year, Stern introduced the resectoscope (Bumpus 1926; Stern 1926).

Approximately 40 years later Keitzer constructed a small cold cutting knife to fit the universal resectoscope and in 1961 and 1969 he published papers on transurethral incision of the bladder neck for contracture (Keitzer et al. 1961, 1969). Orandi published his first results on (*transurethral incision of the prostate* in 1973 (Orandi 1973). At this time, Shafik introduced an open procedure for the incision of the bladder neck, which was exposed retropubically (Shafik 1973).

Today, TUIP is a well established treatment for infravesical obstruction.

Indications for Transurethral Incision of the Prostate

The indications for therapeutic intervention in patients with benign prostatic hyperplasia (BPH) are urinary retention, azotemia with hydronephrosis, gross hematuria, urinary tract infection, overflow incontinence, symptoms of infravesical obstruction, and obstructive urodynamic and cystoscopic findings. Often a patient will present with several of these manifestations of BPH.

The fact that several choices of treatment exist has to be discussed with the patient. He should be encouraged to participate in the selection of treatment. Severe mental disturbance and decreased life expectancy because of comorbid disease are the only strong contraindications to surgery. When the patient has been assigned to prostatic surgery, however, one has to keep in mind that this procedure generally precludes alternative treatment.

Indications for incision and resection of the prostate are nearly equal. Transurethral resection of the prostate (TURP), however, would be preferable to the incision in BPH patients with: (a) symptoms of infravesical obstruction, and larger prostate glands (estimated resectable weight >20–30 g), (b) severe recurrent gross hematuria, and (c) prostatitis, when the aim is to remove the infected prostatic tissue. In younger and/or sexually active BPH patients, the incision technique should preferentially be performed because of the increased incidence of retrograde ejaculation after TURP.

Urodynamic studies are mostly performed to confirm the clinical impression, but also to evaluate parameters that might alter diagnosis or treatments. Symptoms correlate poorly with more objective findings of urinary obstructions, and only hesitancy and slow stream are significantly correlated to urodynamically demonstrated obstruction (Abrams and Feneley 1978).

Surgical Technique

A variety of different instruments have been used in the incision of the bladder neck and prostate including Colling's, Orandi's, and Sach's knife, the standard resectoscope, and Bunt's electrode. Recently the neodymium-yttrium aluminum garnet (Nd-YAG) laser has been introduced to make straightaway incisions or for use in the transurethral ultrasound-guided laser-induced prostatectomy procedure (TULIP).

The primary goal of this procedure is to cut tissue permanently and prevent recurrent obstruction. At the level of the bladder neck the incision is made through the circularly arranged muscle fibers until the urothelium separates widely. The incision is extended distally and deepened through the prostatic adenoma down to and through the prostatic capsule. The bladder neck usually springs apart following this incision. The incision can be performed unilaterally or bilaterally and at a variety of locations around the bladder neck:

1. 12 o'clock (D'Ancona et al. 1990)
2. 10 o'clock (Jenkins and Allen 1978)
3. 9 and 3 o'clock (Loughlin et al. 1987)
4. 4 or/and 8 o'clock (Turner-Warwick et al. 1973; Delaere et al. 1983; Christensen 1985; Hedlund and Ek 1985; Li and Ng 1987; Kelly et al. 1989)

5. 4 or 5 and 7 or 8 o'clock (Andersen et al. 1980)
6. 5 or/and 7 o'clock (Orandi 1973, 1987; Edwards and Powell 1982; Edwards et al. 1985; Moisey et al. 1982; Hellstrom et al. 1986; Dørflinger et al. 1987; Mobb and Moisey 1988; Nielsen 1988; Waymont et al. 1989)
7. 6 o'clock (Graversen et al. 1987; Bruskewitz and Christensen 1990; Katz et al. 1990)

The variety of complications after the incision reflect the complications after any transurethral procedure. They include bleeding, infection, scarring and stricture formation, though the latter condition very seldom results in bladder neck contracture. Retrograde ejaculation is another complication to the transurethral incision and especially to the resection technique.

Results

The evaluation of the efficacy of the treatment of symptomatic BPH patients, or patients suffering from any other disease, is often compromised by the failure to objectify patients' subjective symptoms. Use of symptom scoring schemes such as proposed by Madsen (Madsen and Iversen 1983) or Boyarsky (Boyarsky et al. 1977) minimize some of the uncertainty about subjective symptoms in BPH patients. Also, one has to keep in mind that more than 30% of men with untreated symptomatic BPH will experience regression in subjective symptoms and more than 20% will show regression in objective criteria for urinary obstruction when followed over approximately 2.5–5 years (Isaacs 1990).

The best studies are those which compare the efficacy of two procedures by randomizing patients to one or the other. By such randomization the potential bias in assigning a patient to one treatment or another is avoided.

Horan randomized patients to either balloon dilatation or incision of the prostate and showed that all patients in the incision group had regression in voiding symptoms compared to 66% in the balloon dilatation group (follow-up unstated) (Horan et al. 1990). Li and Ng (1987), Larsen et al. (1987), Dørflinger et al. (1987), Nielsen (1988), and Christensen et al. (1990) have been the first to publish the results of studies in which patients were randomized to either TUIP or TURP. The results are shown in Tables 1–3. In the study of Li and Ng, preoperative flows or analysis of symptoms are not stated.

The conclusion of these studies is that incision of the prostate and bladder neck relieves urinary outflow obstruction, as does TURP. The postoperative peak flow in the TURP group is slightly higher than in the TUIP group, and possibly symptom relief is a little better in the TURP group as well. These statements on flow and subjective symptoms, however, are only based on four and three trials, respectively. The incidence of retrograde ejaculation in these randomized studies on average reflects the results found in other studies (Riehmann and Bruskewitz 1991).

Table 1. Results of randomized studies: peak flow (ml/s)

	TUIP		TURP	
	Preoperative	*Postoperative*	*Preoperative*	*Postoperative*
Dorflinger et al. 1987	10.0	15.0	9.0	19.0
Larsen et al. 1987	7.4	14.4	8.6	16.3
Nielsen 1988	5.0	10.0	5.0	17.0
Christensen et al. 1990	7.8	12.7	9.7	16.6
Mean ~	8	13	8	17

Table 2. Results of randomized studies: change (%) in subjective symptoms

	TUIP			TURP		
	Better	*No change*	*Worse*	*Better*	*No change*	*Worse*
Dorflinger et al. 1987	93	7		95	5	
Larsen et al. 1987	95	5		94	6	
Christensen et al. 1990	81		19[a]	95		5[a]
Mean ~	90			95		

[a]same + worse

Table 3. Results of randomized studies: retrograde ejaculation (%)

	TUIP	TURP
Dorflinger et al. 1987	0	45
Larsen et al. 1987	28	100
Christensen 1990	13	37
Mean ~	14	61

Nielsen found a significantly shorter operative time in the incision group than in the TURP group (Nielsen 1988). Li found the operative time for TUIP to be about half the time required for resection, but this difference was not statistically significant in their small study (Li and Ng 1987). Reduced operative time minimizes the fluid absorption which is problematic with TURP (Li and Ng 1987). It may also decrease the incidence of postoperative pulmonary and cardiovascular complications. Dørflinger found significantly lower operative time and blood loss during surgery in favor of the TUIP group (Dørflinger et al. 1987). Compared to TURP, the incision is, in addition, relatively simple to perform and teach. Under the correct indications this procedure is a very good alternative to TURP.

From TUIP/TURP nonrandomized matched studies it is known that the incision technique, as the sole primary procedure, should be reserved for smaller glands because of increased difficulty and increased incidence of complications when larger glands are incised (Orandi 1987; Edwards 1989). Symptom relief, however, is also less often seen when larger glands are incised.

Cost-Saving Advantages of Transurethral Incision of the Prostate

Postoperative stay after TUIP is about 2 days shorter than after transurethral resection (Li and Ng 1987; Edwards 1989). The incision can also more easily be performed under local anesthesia (Loughlin et al. 1987; Graversen et al. 1987). These conditions together with reduced operative time and decreased perioperative morbidity make TUIP potentially less expensive.

Bladder Neck Contracture

Approximately 8% of the TURP patients develop bladder neck contraction after surgery in smaller glands, but this is very seldom seen after incision of the prostate (Sikafi et al. 1985; Mebust 1987; Orandi 1990). Postresection vesical neck contracture following TURP is generally treated with bladder neck incision (Sikafi et al. 1985). By performing prophylactic bladder neck incision in conjunction with TURP in smaller glands (estimated resected weight of <20 g), the incidence of bladder neck contracture is reduced to about 1% (Kulb et al. 1987).

Prostate Cancer Risk

The disadvantage of TUIP is the potential for missing stage A prostatic cancer. In the elderly population, the missed diagnosis of prostate cancer stage A might not be of major importance, but in the younger it could lead to reduced survival.

   Prostate-specific antigen (PSA) and transurethral ultrasonography are options to increase the early detection of prostatic cancer, but thus far neither of these screening methods nor digital rectal examination have been shown to significantly decrease mortality (Chodak 1989). In order to obtain some tissue for histological examination, the resectoscope loop could be used to perform the "incision" or one could do a simultaneous needle biopsy.

Conclusions

Transurethral incision of the prostate and bladder neck relieves Urinary outflow obstruction as does TURP among patients randomized to these procedures. There are, however, some important differences in both the outcome and the indications for these two procedures.

   The incision technique should only be performed in men with glands of an estimated resected weight of <20 g because of poorer postoperative outcome and increased complication rate when the procedure is performed in men with larger prostate glands. The incision should preferentially be performed in younger or sexually active men because the incidence of retrograde ejaculation is 40%–50% lower than after TURP. TUIP is: (a) relatively easy to learn and perform, (b) associated with a shorter operative time, and hospital stay and (c) accompanied by decreased blood loss during surgery and perioperative morbidity compared to TURP. Thus, TUIP is potentially less expensive than TURP.

A disadvantage of the incision technique, however, is the possibility of missing occult prostatic cancer. This could, to some extent, be overcome by using the resectoscope loop to perform the "incision" or doing a simultaneous needle biopsy.

References

Abrams PH, Feneley RCL (1978) The significance of the symptoms associated with bladder outflow obstruction. Urol Int 33:171–174

Andersen JT, Nordling J, Meyhoff HH, Jacobsen O, Hald, T (1980) Functional bladder neck obstruction: late results after endoscopic bladder neck incision. Scand J Urol Nephrol 14:17–22

Blain D (1983) Transurethral prostatic resection. Technique of T.M. Davis. Urology 21:93–101

Boyarsky S, Jones G, Paulson DF, Prout GR (1977) A new look at bladder neck obstruction by the Food and Drug Administration regulators: guidelines for investigation of benign prostatic hypertrophy. Trans Am Assoc, Genito Urinary Surg 68:29–32

Bruskewitz RC, Christensen MM (1990) Critical evaluation of transurethral resection and incision of the prostate. Prostate Suppl 3:27–28

Bumpus HC (1926) Results of punch prostatectomy. J Urol 16:59–66

Chodak GW (1989) Early detection and screening for prostatic cancer. Urology [Suppl] 34(4):10–12

Christensen MG, Nordling J, Andersen JT, Hald T (1985) Functional bladder neck obstruction. Results of endoscopic bladder neck incision in 131 consecutive patients. Br J Urol 57:60–62

Christensen MM, Aagaard J, Madsen PO (1990) Transurethral resection versus transurethral incision of the prostate. Urol Clin North Am 17(3):621–630

D'Ancona CAL, Netto NR Jr, Cara AM, Ikari O (1990) Internal urethrotomy of the prostatic urethra or transurethral resection in benign prostatic hyperplasia. J Urol 144:918–920

Delaere KPJ, Debruyne FMJ, Moonen WA (1983) Extended bladder neck incision for outflow obstruction inmale patients. Br J Urol 55:225–228

Dørflinger T, Øster M, Larsen JF, Walter S, Krarup T (1987) Transurethral prostatectomy or incision of the prostate in the treatment of prostatism caused by small benign prostates. Scand J Urol Nephrol 104:77–81

Edwards L, Powell C (1982) An objective comparison of transurethral resection and bladder neck incision in the treatment of prostatic hypertrophy. J Urol 128:325–327

Edwards LE (1989) Transurethral incision of the prostate or bladder neck incision. In: Fitzpatrick JM, Krane RJ (eds) The prostate. Livingstone, Edinburgh, pp 245–249

Edwards LE, Bucknall TE, Pittman MR, Richardson DR, Stanek J (1985) Transurethral resection of the prostate and bladder neck incision: a review of 700 cases. Br J Urol 57:168–171

Graversen PH, Gasser TC, Larsen EH, Dørflinger T, Bruskewitz RC (1987) Transurethral incisions of the prostate under local anesthesia in high-risk patients: a pilot study. Scand J Urol 104:87–90

Hedlund H, Ek A (1985) Ejaculation and sexual function after endoscopic bladder neck incision. Br J Urol 57:164–167

Hellstrom P, Lukkarinen O, Kontturi M (1986) Bladder neck incision or transurethral electroresection for the treatment of urinary obstruction caused by a small benign prostate? A randomized urodynamic study. Scand J Urol Nephrol 20:187–192

Horan JJ, Chiou RK, Binard JE, Ebersole ME, Dunne EF (1990) Balloon dilatation of prostate: a randomized study comparing with transurethral incision of prostate. J Urol 143:281A

Isaacs JT (1990) Importance of the natural history of benign prostatic hyperplasia in the evaluation of pharmacologic intervention. Prostate Suppl 3:1–7

Jenkins JD, Allen NH (1978) Bladder neck incision–a treatment for retention with overflow in the absence of adenoma. Br J Urol 50:395–397

Katz PG, Greenstein A, Ratliff JE, Marks S, Guice J (1990) Transurethral incision of the bladder neck and prostate. J Urol 144:694–696

Keitzer WA, Cervantes L, Demaculangan A, Cruz B (1961) Transurethral incision of bladder neck for contracture. J Urol 86:242–246

Keitzer WA, Tandon B, Allen J, Bernreuter E, Amador J (1969) Urethrotomy visualized for bladder neck contracture in male patients. J Urol 102:577–580

Kelly MJ, Roskamp D, Leach GE (1989) Transurethral incision of the prostate: a preoperative and postoperative analysis of symptoms and urodynamic findings. J Urol 142:1507–1509

Kulb TB, Kamer M, Lingeman JE, Foster RS (1987) Prevention of post-prostatectomy vesical neck contracture by prophylactic vesical neck incision. J Urol 137:230–231

Larsen EH, Dørflinger T, Gasser TC, Graversen PH, Bruskewitz RC (1987) Transurethral incision versus transurethral resection of the prostate for the treatment of benign prostatic hypertrophy. A preliminary report. Scand J Urol Nephrol 104:83–86

Li MK, Ng SM (1987) Bladder neck resection and transurethral resection of the prostate: a randomized prospective trial. J Urol 138:807–809

Loughlin KR, Yalla SV, Belldegrun A, Berstein GT (1987) Transurethral incisions and resections under local anesthesia. Br J Urol 60:185

Madsen PO, Iversen P (1983) A point system for selecting operative candidates. In: Hinman F (ed) Benign Prostatic Hypertrophy. Springer, Berlin Heidelberg New York, pp 763–765

Mebust WK (1987) Transurethral incision or resection of the prostate. J Urol 138:852

Mobb GE, Moisey CU (1988) Long-term follow-up of unilateral bladder neck incision. Br J Urol 62:160–162

Moisey CU, Stephenson TP, Evans C (1982) A subjective and urodynamic assessment of unilateral bladder neck incision for bladder neck obstruction. Br J Urol 54:114–117

Nielsen HO (1988) Transurethral prostatotomy versus transurethral prostatectomy in benign prostatic hypertrophy. A prospective randomized study. Br J Urol 61:435–438

Orandi A (1973) Transurethral incision of the prostate. J Urol 110:229–231

Orandi A (1987) Transurethral incision of prostate compared with transurethral resection of prostate in 132 matching cases. J Urol 138:810–815

Orandi A (1990) Transurethral resection versus transurethral incision of the prostate. Urol Clin North Am 17(3):601–612

Riehmann M, Bruskewitz R (1991) Transurethral incision of the prostate (TUIP) and bladder neck. J Androl 12:415–422

Shafik A (1973) Cystomyotomy: a technique for the cure of bladder neck obstruction. J Urol 110:657–659

Shelley HS (1969) The enlarged prostate: a brief history of its treatment. J Hist Med Allied Sci 24:452–473

Sikafi Z, Butler MR, Lane V, O'Flynn JD, Fitzpatrick JM (1985) Bladder neck contracture following prostatectomy. Br J Urol 57:308–310

Stern M (1926) Resection of obstructions at the vesical orifice: new instruments and a new method. JAMA 87:1726–1730

Turner-Warwick R, Whiteside CG, Worth PHL, Milroy EJG, Bates CP (1973) A urodynamic view of the clinical problems associated with bladder neck dysfunction and its treatment by endoscopic incision and trans-trigonal posterior prostatectomy. Br J Urol 45:44–59

Waymont B, Ward JP, Perry KC (1989) Long-term assessment of 107 patients undergoing bladder neck incision. Br J Urol 64:280–282

Young HH (1913) A new procedure (punch operation) for small prostatic bars and contracture of the prostatic orifice. JAMA 60:253–257

Balloon Dilatation of the Prostate

S.L.Goldenberg

Introduction

An emergence of interest in medical and surgical alternatives to the classic transurethral prostatectomy has occurred in the last decade. These treatments are aimed at the static and dynamic components of infravesical obstruction (Caine 1986). Transurethral prostatic resection eliminates static obstructing tissue and is a reliable and effective operation in most patients, especially those with larger glands. In men with minimal prostate enlargement or "primary bladder neck hyperplasia," the dynamic neurologically mediated component is prominent, and these individuals may respond well to alternative therapies. One specific type of medical therapy involves α-adrenergic blocking agents. This chapter reviews the current status of another alternative, balloon dilatation of the prostate, which affects both the static and dynamic obstructive factors.

In the past few years numerous centers have evaluated balloon dilatation of the prostate. There are now multiple technical variations, diverse reports on the subjective and objective responses, and much speculation on the mechanisms of action. Early investigators used fluoroscopically placed balloons. Subsequently, systems utilizing digitally directed placement methods, ultrasound-guided positioning, and endoscopic techniques have been introduced. Balloons are now available in sizes of 75F, 90F, or 105F and come in single length or "sized-to-fit" length systems.

The early enthusiasm towards balloon dilation has matured into a "cautious assessment" attitude, as investigators attempt to find its place in the urologist's armamentarium. It is possible to identify subgroups of patients that clearly benefit from balloon dilatation. Much work remains to be done to better define this "ideal" candidate, to determine the mechanism of action in order to modify the techniques accordingly and optimize results. It is becoming clear that balloon dilatation is not a substitute in an appropriate situation for transurethral resection any more than transurethral resection is a substitute for open enucleation.

Historical Perspective

Like most things in medicine, dilatation of the prostate is not new. In fact, mechanical dilatation of the prostatic urethra was first performed in the mid-nineteenth century! In 1910, transvesical digital dilatation of the prostate was described by Hollingsworth (1910). The concept of relieving infravesical obstruction by transvesical anterior and posterior commissurotomies (with maintenance of sexual functioning) was proposed by Franck in 1938 (Deisting 1956). This idea was applied to a transurethral approach by Deisting in 1956. He reported his results in 324 patients dilated with an instrument resembling a reverse-action forceps (Deisting 1956). Deisting stated that his dilatation results compared favorably with a simultaneous series of suprapubic prostatectomies. In addition to commissurotomy, he theorized that prolonged dilatation exhausted the elasticity of the prostatic capsule. In 1963, Karl-Axel Backman reported on his 2 year experience with the Deisting forcep (Backman 1963). Though his patients did well for 1 year, their symptoms deteriorated during the second year of follow-up. In a double-arm study Aalkjaer compared Deisting dilatation to standard prostatectomy (Aalkjaer 1965). He found that the dilatation method "will have a certain modest favourable effect on the bladder emptying conditions in some cases" but prostatectomy "will render far better immediate results with less postoperative complications" and statistically significant better results up to 7 years postoperatively.

In 1974 Gruntzig and Hopff popularized the use of a balloon dilation catheter for the nonoperative relief of vascular obstruction (Backman 1963). In 1984, H.J. Burhenne was the first to apply the modern balloon dilatation technique to the prostate (his own!) (Burhenne et al. 1984). Subsequent, preliminary human clinical trials reported "success" rates ranging from 47% to 91%, with minimal complications (Burhenne et al. 1984; Castaneda et al. 1987; Quinn et al. 1985; Reddy et al. 1987; Sandberg and Sandstrom 1967).

The Balloons

Single Length, Single Balloon

The first catheter dilatations were performed using fluoroscopic guidance to place the dilating balloon proximal to the external sphincter (Reddy et al. 1987). The single balloon catheter is 40 cm long and can be inflated to a diameter of 75F (Medi-Tech, Inc., Watertown, MA; shown in Fig. 1). At full inflation, it exerts three atmospheres of pressure against the surrounding prostate tissue. A retrograde urethrogram is done to locate the proximal end of the external sphincter and this site is marked by pinning a needle to overlying drapes. The balloon is passed over a 0.038-inch guide wire and is positioned with the radiopaque marker at the level of the external sphincter.

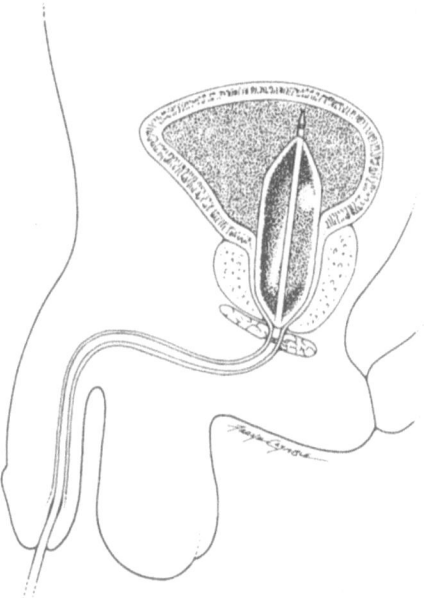

Fig. 1. Medi-Tech single length, single balloon catheter (Watertown, MA), 40 cm long and inflated to a diameter of 75F, passed into the bladder over a 0.038-inch guidewire under fluoroscopic guidance

One shortcoming of this technique is the inability to precisely identify the external sphincter, potentially resulting in dilatation through the sphincter if the catheter is positioned too distal. If, however, the balloon is placed too proximal to the sphincter then the full length of the prostatic urethra will not be dilated. Another drawback of fluoroscopic placement of the single length balloon is its tendency to migrate into the bladder during the inflation procedure (Fig. 2). With initial filling, the intravesical portion of the balloon, which has no external pressure applied to it, selectively inflates and pulls the catheter forward into the bladder. To overcome this migration it is necessary to apply firm countertraction to the catheter, which further diminishes the accuracy of placement.

Single Length, Double Balloons

The next generation of single length balloon incorporated a second proximal ("locating") balloon 1.5 cm proximal to the dilating balloon on the catheter shaft (Optilume, American Medical Systems, Minnetonka, MN; shown in Fig. 3). As with the single balloon catheter, these two balloons are delineated by radiopaque markers allowing fluoroscopic placement. There is also a firm positioning collar at the proximal end of the dilating balloon which can be palpated transrectally, offering a digital positioning option.

After the catheter is passed over a 0.038-inch guide wire into the bladder, the locating balloon is filled with 0.5 ml of water. The catheter is withdrawn until this balloon is felt to "pop" through the sphincter. The positioning collar should be palpable at the apex of the gland and held in that position while the locating

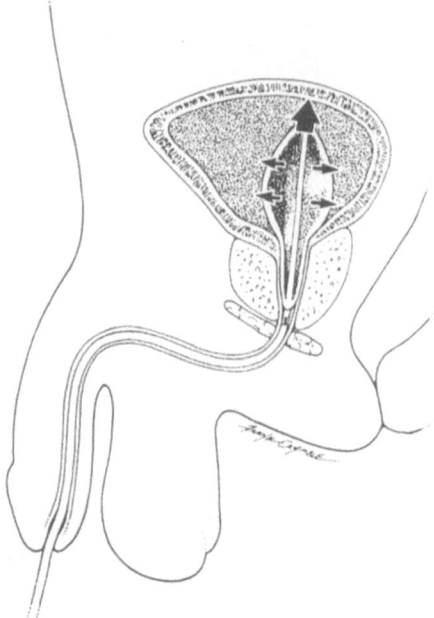

Fig. 2. Single length dilatation balloons inflate in the bladder before inflating in the prostatic urethra. Retropropagation of the inflation draws the balloon into the bladder ("migration")

balloon is inflated to its capacity of 1.5 ml (40F) in the bulbous urethra. This is intended to fix the catheter in place, to reduce the migration problem, and assure dilatation of the prostatic apex.

The dilating balloon is 4 cm long, tapers through the bladder neck portion, and can be inflated to a maximum diameter of 90F with a pressure of 4 atm (60 psi).

Single Length, Palpating Nodule

A third type of single length balloon catheter has been designed with a 24F palpating button or nodule 5 mm proximal to the dilating balloon (Dowd II, Microvasive, Boston Scientific Corp., Watertown, MA; shown in Fig. 4). This facilitates transrectal digital positioning of the catheter at the apex of the gland. The dilatation catheter is advanced into the bladder over a 0.038 inch guidewire and is withdrawn until the positioning nodule is palpable just beyond the apex of the gland. It is held at this position by the rectal digit while the balloon is fully inflated to a diameter of 90F at a pressure of 4 atm (60 psi). The catheter has a unique collar on the external part of the catheter to allow countertraction but migration can still be a problem. Personally, I have found it difficult to accurately maintain the position of this balloon as the nodule becomes more difficult to palpate with certainty when the compressed prostate tissue is forced outwards towards the

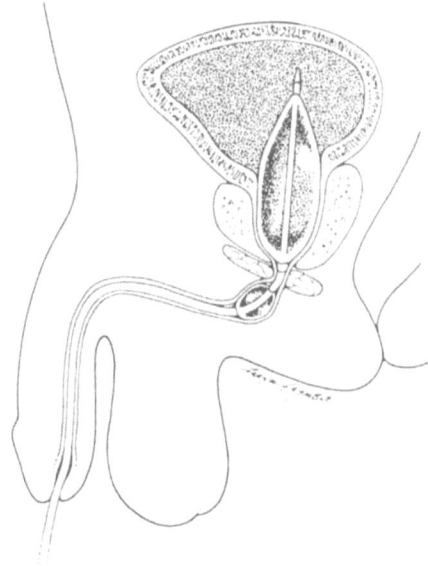

Fig. 3. Single length balloon incorporating a second proximal ("locating") balloon into the catheter. This locating balloon (1.5 ml, 40F) is situated 1.5 cm proximal to the dilating balloon and is intended to fix the catheter in place. The dilating balloon is 4 cm long and can be inflated to a maximum diameter of 90F. The firm collar can be palpated transrectally and positioned at the prostatic apex. (Optilume, American Medical Systems, Minnetonka, MN)

membranous urethra. Transrectal ultrasound (TRUS) shows that this occurs without the full length of the prostate being dilated. If this occurs the balloon should be deflated and repositioned with firm countertraction applied throughout the dilating process (see below).

Digitally guided techniques are generally subjective, blind, and dependent on the operator's experience and judgement. For these reasons, visual endoscopic or ultrasound-guided placement techniques have been developed.

Sized-To-Fit Balloon

In 1988, Klein reported on a transcystoscopic method of balloon placement (Klein and Leeming 1988). With this system (Uroplasty, Advanced Surgical Intervention (ASI), San Clemente, CA), the length of the prostatic urethra is measured from bladder neck to external sphincter and the appropriate "sized-to-fit" balloon catheter is precisely positioned proximal to the external sphincter. The position of the ballon is endoscopically monitored throughout the inflation process and one can be confident of a full length prostatic urethral dilatation without migration. The ASI balloon is either 75F or 90F in diameter, inflates to a pressure of 4 atm, and is available in effective dilating lengths of 1.5–4.0 cm.

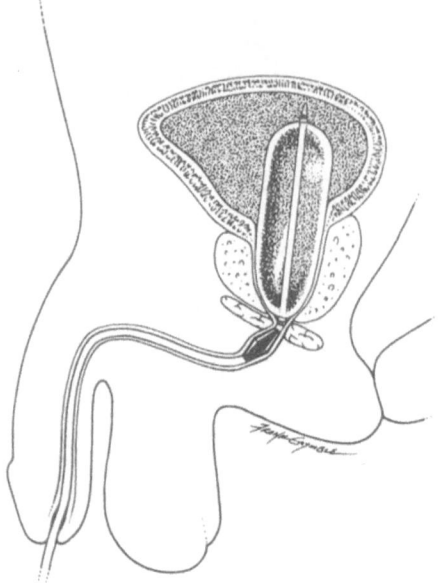

Fig. 4. Single length ballon with a 24F palpating button or nodule 5 mm proximal to the dilating balloon, for transrectal digital positioning of the catheter at the apex of the gland. When fully inflated the balloon achieves a diameter of 90F. A unique traction collar on the external part of the catheter (not shown) counters the effect of catheter migration. (Dowd II, Microvasive, Boston Scientific Corp., Watertown, MA)

Ultrasound-Guided Dilatation

If one has a TRUS probe available in the cystoscopy suite, then any one of the balloon systems can be placed using ultrasound guidance. The balloon can first be positioned by digital or cystoscopic control and TRUS can then be used to confirm the balloon's position relative to the prostate apex (it is particularly reassuring to be able to visualize the dilated balloon extending right down to the level of, but not through, the external sphincter). Incorporating TRUS into the procedure makes it more cumbersome but, with some practice, it is easily integrated and certainly adds to its precision, safety, and ultimate clinical success. Ultrasound findings are further discussed below.

Preoperative Evaluation

Prior to balloon dilatation all patients are evaluated as they would be for a transurethral resection or any other therapeutic procedure directed at prostatic obstruction. In the earlier days of this procedure, many of the subjects were chosen only because they were too ill to withstand a transurethral prostatectomy. This proved to be a poor reason to proceed as most of these men were carrying high residuals with large glands or were in total urinary retention. Not surprisingly, the majority failed to respond satisfactorily to balloon dilatation.

One should take a full history of obstructive and irritative symptoms. This is facilitated by the use of a semiquantitative and reasonably objective scoring system (eg. Boyarsky, Madsen, WHO). Routine hematology, urinalysis, urine culture, and blood chemistry are also obtained. A careful digital rectal examination should be performed and if cancer is suspected one should draw blood for prostate-specific antigen (and/or acid phosphatase) and proceed to TRUS with guided biopsies.

All potential balloon candidates should be screened with uroflowmetry and residual urine determination by catheter or ultrasound scan. This simple screen will help detect patients with decompensated bladders (residual urine of more than 50% of bladder capacity) and those with normal flow rates and residuals who are not likely to benefit from dilatation and require further investigations. Although there are sophisticated urodynamic studies to diagnose outflow tract obstruction (e.g., pressure-flow nomograms) these have not gained wide acceptance nor have they proven to be clinically relevant. They may be useful, however, in evaluating complex or borderline cases.

Radiological studies such as retrograde urethrography and voiding cystography do not either predict or correlate with clinical improvement (Reddy et al. 1988) and are not recommended.

The decision to proceed to balloon dilatation is ultimately made at cystoscopy. It is important to rule out urethral stricture, meatal stenosis, middle lobe hypertrophy, or an extremely large prostate, all of which are clear contraindications to this form of treatment. All patients should receive perioperative antibiotic therapy and urine cultures must be clear prior to the procedure.

Transurethral balloon dilatation may be carried out under any form of anesthesia. It has been reportedly done under topical anesthesia with intravenous sedation. My experience has been that these patients have a lot of bladder spasms which interferes with the performance of the procedure. Reddy has described a periprostatic nerve block (Reddy et al. 1988). This can be somewhat tedious, time-consuming and not always reliable (particularly in large men), often requiring substantial adjunctive intravenous medication. A spinal anesthestic provides excellent intraoperative and early postoperative pain and spasm control. Patients tend to have most of these bladder spasms within the first 3–4 h following dilatation. Once the spinal wears off, the spasms tend to be a minor problem and are manageable with anticholinergic medications. I believe that the spinal (regional) is the anesthetic of choice for balloon dilatation.

Technique of Endoscopic Balloon Dilatation

A calibration catheter is placed through the cystoscope working channel to determine the length, in centimeters, of the prostatic urethra from bladder neck to external sphincter (Fig. 5). A 26F balloon system sheath is then passed into the

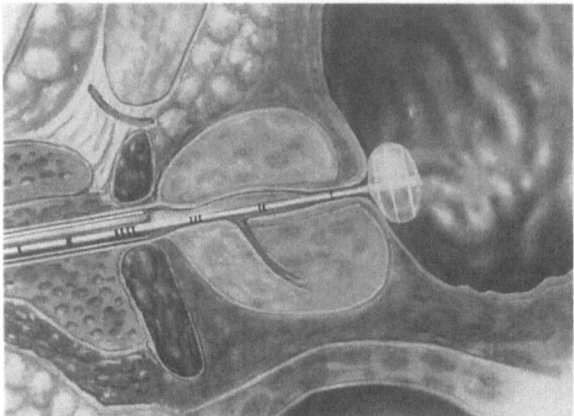

Fig. 5. Urethral calibration catheter positioned in prostatic urethra with inflated balloon against bladder neck. The anatomical length of the urethra is determined using the cm markings on the catheter shaft. (Uroplasty, Advanced Surgical Intervention, San Clemente, CA)

bladder and a well lubricated, appropriately sized, dilatation catheter is advanced through the sheath. A key element of the dilating catheter is the Foley balloon which is inflated in the bladder and then snugged down against the bladder neck (Fig. 6). This positions the dilating balloon in the prostatic urethra. Confirmation of this position and further "fine-tuning" is done by visually placing a white localization line (0.5 cm from the dilating balloon) just outside of the sphincter (Figs. 6, 7). By placing this line distal to the sphincter one can be sure of dilating the prostatic apex. If the localization line is placed proximal to this location (a common error is placing it at the verumontanum) then there will be a tendency for migration into

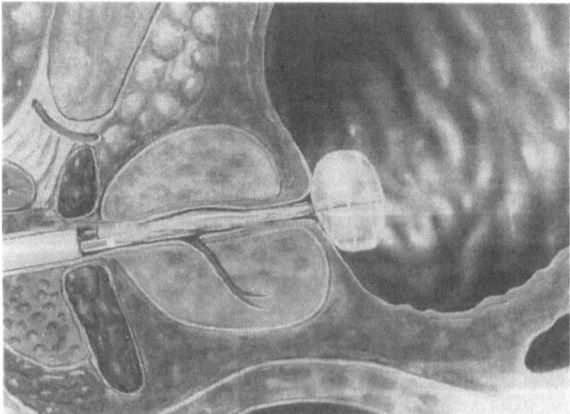

Fig. 6. Dilatation balloon in prostatic urethra with Foley balloon pulled back against the bladder neck. The white line is endoscopically positioned at the external sphincter. (Uroplasty, Advanced Surgical Intervention, San Clemente, CA)

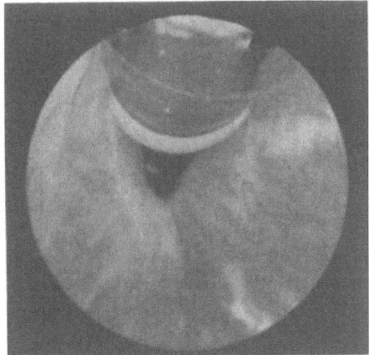

Fig. 7. Cystoscopic appearance of the white line on the catheter positioned just distal to the external sphincter

the bladder as the balloon inflates across the bladder neck. While endoscopically ensuring that the white line remains in its position in the bulbous urethra, the dilatation balloon is inflated by an assistant using a hand-held positive displacement pump with integral pressure gauge. Occasionally, during the initial inflation, the catheter tends to displace towards the bladder. With the Uroplasty system only mild traction is needed for a few seconds to overcome this tendency. Once the sized-to-fit balloon is fully inflated it will sit in the prostatic fossa and will not be able to be displaced proximally or distally, even with forced traction (Fig. 8).

As the prostate capsule stretches, the pressure gauge will indicate a drop in pressure requiring the addition of more fluid to the balloon until the inflating pressure is restored. Dilatation is maintained for at least 10 min after which the deflated catheter is withdrawn through its sheath as a single unit, minimizing the trauma to the distal urethra.

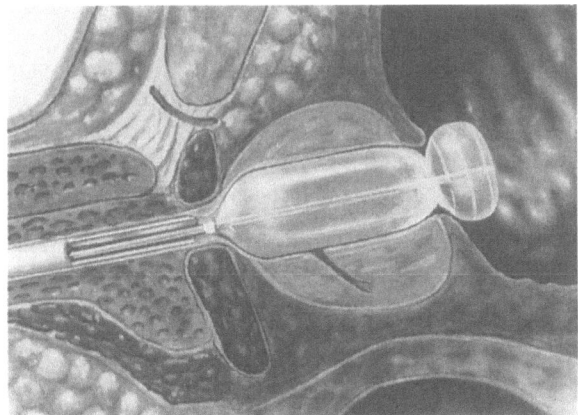

Fig. 8. The sized-to-fit dilatation balloon shown inflating the entire prostatic urethra from bladder neck to apex. Note that the bladder neck is only partially stretched and not fully dilated. (Uroplasty, Advanced Surgical Intervention, San Clemente, CA)

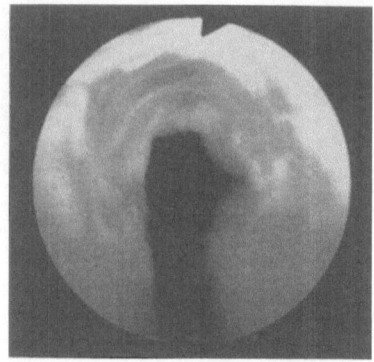

Fig. 9. Cystoscopic view of the anterior commissurotomy created by balloon dilatation of the prostate

At the completion of the procedure, the cystoscope should be reintroduced and
the prostatic fossa carefully examined. If adequate dilatation has been achieved
there should be a mucosal tear extending from just distal to the bladder neck
towards the apex, usually in the anterior commissure (Fig. 9). There will often
be small bleeding vessels which rarely require fulguration. Any clots which have
collected in the bladder should be evacuated with a Toomey syringe and then a 20F
or 22F irrigating catheter placed on continuous saline irrigations. These irrigations
are continued until clear, usually for 6–8 h.

Postoperative Care

The catheter is left in place for a minimum of 48 h on an outpatient basis. Patients
should be warned that they may see bleeding around the Foley catheter from the
meatus and once the catheter has been removed minor hematuria may continue
for several days. It is most unusual for this to result in clot retention. All of my
patients have been treated with perioperative antibiotics and infection has not been
a problem.

Patients should not expect to feel significant improvement immediately upon
removal of the catheter. As with a prostatectomy, relief is often not experienced
until the urothelium repairs. It often takes 3 months to attain maximum relief of
symptoms. No urologist would recommend a repeat prostatectomy for ongoing
symptoms soon after the primary resection, and the same is true following balloon
dilatation. My patients are seen at 3, 6, 12, 18, and 24 months follow-up, with
symptom score evaluation, flow rates, and postvoid residual determinations.

Mechanism of Action

The exact mechanism by which balloon dilatation of the prostate improves voiding
is not well understood. It may affect either, or both, the static and dynamic compo-

nents of obstruction. The application of an extremely high pressure (five times the pressure of the Deisting dilator) by a noncompliant balloon to the posterior urethra leads to stretching of the prostate capsule with compression and divulsion of the prostatic lobes. The anterior commissurotomy has been well documented in canine studies and in human investigations utilizing the prostates of living organ donors (Goldenberg and Perez-Marerro 1992) (Fig. 10). Whether or not it helps to resolve urinary symptoms is unclear but it is important to cystoscopically observe this tear as an indicator of adequate dilatation. The "sized-to-fit" balloon does not split through the bladder neck and this explains why antegrade ejaculation is always maintained with this system.

In our first group of patients we measured serum prostate-specific antigen (PSA) levels immediately before and after dilatation (Goldenberg et al. 1990). We found that serum PSA increased by greater than 1.5 ng/ml in 16/22 patients and in all patients returned to predilatation levels within 3 months. This observation also supports the concept of mechanical disruption of the prostate by balloon dilatation.

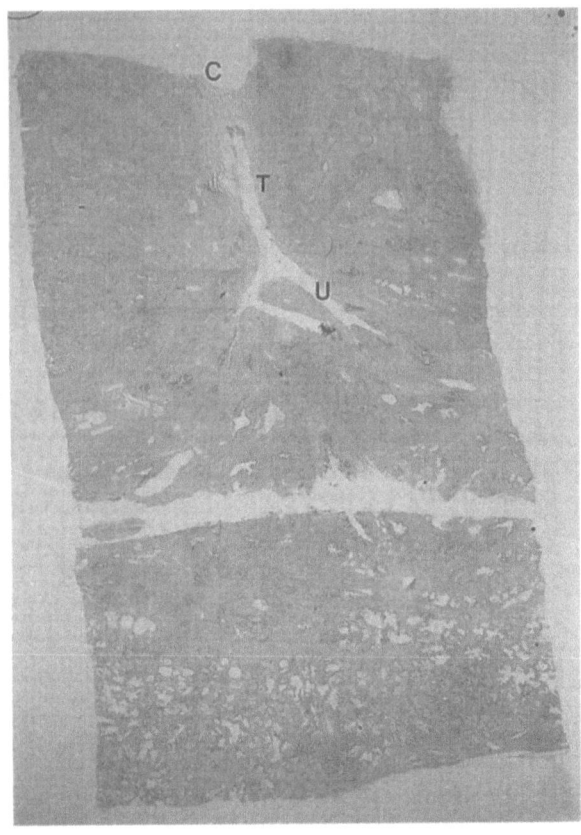

Fig. 10. Transverse section photomicrograph (H&E) showing the anterior tear (T) extending from urethra (U) to the capsule (C)

The dynamic component of obstruction, as defined by Caine (1986), results from the activity of α 1-adrenergic neuroreceptors. These are distributed throughout the bladder neck and prostatic adenoma, particularly within the prostatic capsule, and mediate the contractility of the prostatic urethral smooth muscle. Pharmacologic therapy with α-blockers has been successful in decreasing the tone of prostate smooth muscle and the resistance to outflow with an improvement in symptoms (Lepor 1989).

The full-length compression of the prostate adenoma with expansile stretching of the capsule may alter neuroreceptor distribution and/or function (Fig. 11). This concept would explain the reduction of irritative voiding symptoms in patients who have undergone balloon dilatation. In our experience, patients with "primary" bladder neck hyperplasia or clinical obstruction with a normal-sized prostate responded well to balloon dilatation without endoscopic or radiologic disruption of the bladder neck (Goldenberg et al. 1990). It is possible that the dynamic component was directly affected by capsular distention with an alteration/disruption of neuroreceptor activity. Symptom relief may have also been due to some other, ill-defined mechanism within the prostatic urethra that is unrelated to anatomical obstruction or neuroreceptor activity. I believe that, to optimize the result, it is as important to stretch the entire prostate capsule, from bladder neck to apex, as it is to include the apical tissue in an adequate transurethral prostatectomy. This is perhaps the greatest advantage of the sized-to-fit balloon which guarantees this full length dilatation (see below).

Transrectal Ultrasound Study

Differences between clinical trials may be attributed to the diverse types of balloons and the variability of their effect on the prostate capsule. Undoubtedly, any balloon that can distend to 75 F or 90 F will lead to a mechanical disruption of prostate tissue. However, what may be more important is the achievement of an adequate stretch of the entire prostatic capsule, including the apical region. TRUS allows us to see if, and how, balloon dilatation does this.

I initially used the TRUS probe to measure the volume, area, circumference, and length of prostates before, during, and after dilatation. I then compared the effects of the custom (sized-to-fit) length balloon to the single length balloon systems.

My results confirm that during a 75 F dilatation the capsule stretches with an increase in all measured parameters of at least 22% ($n = 16$), including a 69% increase in glandular volume ($n = 9$). The sized-to-fit balloons (unlike the single length balloons) inflate initially within the prostate and not in the bladder. Also, the sized-to-fit balloon clearly dilates the entire length of the prostatic fossa from bladder neck to apex, sparing the bladder neck (thus the antegrade ejaculation) and sphincter in every case (Fig. 12, 13). During inflation the balloon becomes "encapsulated" within the prostate, maximizing the applied radial forces from apex to base. These forces are mostly applied to the anterior fibromuscular stroma,

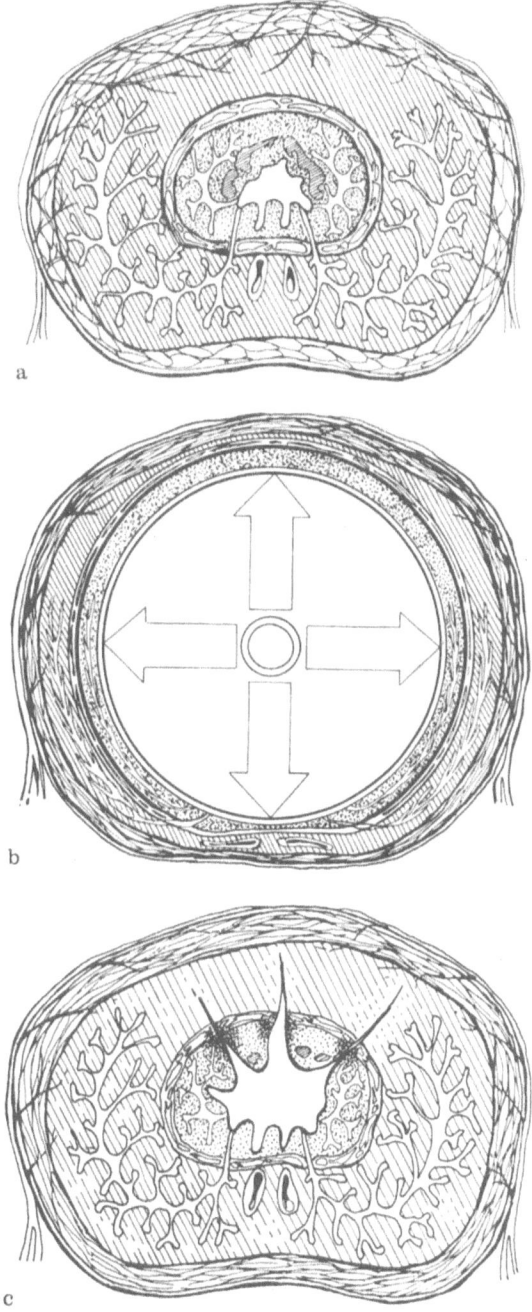

Fig. 11 a – c. During dilatation, compression of the prostate adenoma and expansile stretching of the capsule may alter neuroreceptor distribution and/or function. **a** Undilated gland; **b** during dilatation; **c** following dilatation

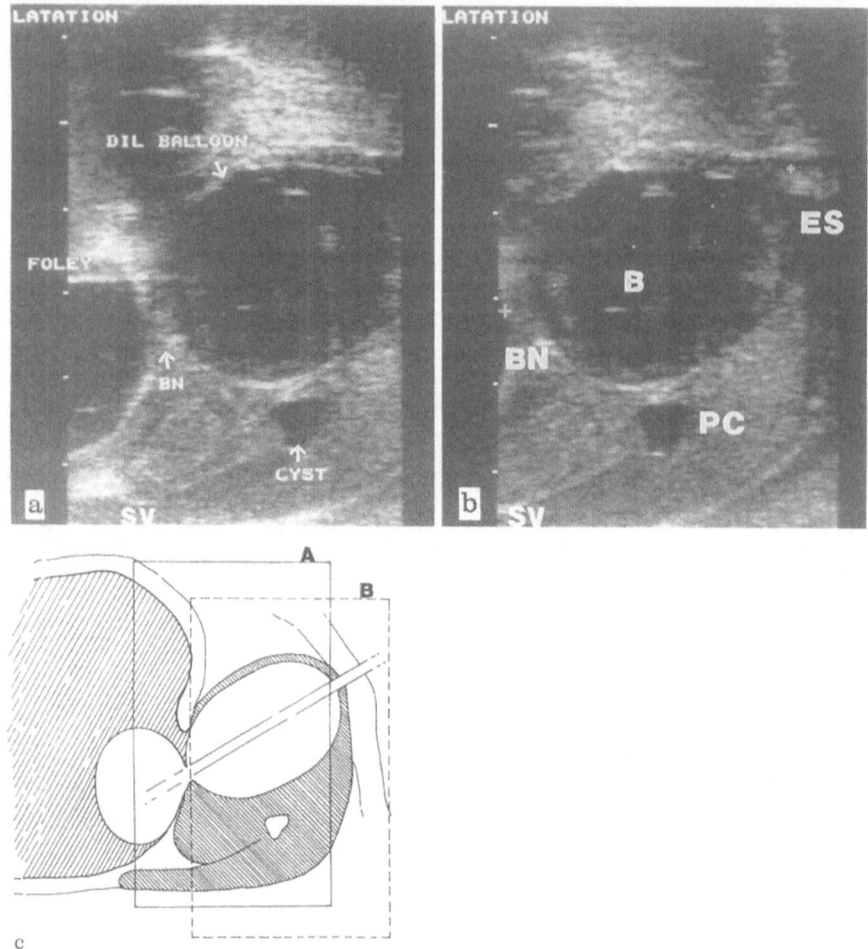

Fig. 12 a – c. Midsaggital transverse transrectal ultrasound (TRUS) scan during dilatation with the ASI Uroplasty catheter. Note how the prostate is being dilated in its entire length from the bladder neck to the external sphincter. (*PC*, prostate cyst; *BN*, bladder neck; *B*, balloon; *ES*, external sphincter; *SV*, seminal vesical). **c** TRUS of *solid line square* (including prostatovesical junction) shown in **a**; TRUS of *dashed line square* (including apical prostate and sphincter) shown in **b**

with very little effect on the peripheral zone, resulting in an anterior tear or commissurotomy (Fig. 14).

In this study, the single length balloon systems, when positioned under digital, fluroscopic, or ultrasound control, always migrated into the bladder upon initial inflation. Even with forceful countertraction, ultrasound showed that the prostate was being dilated only in its proximal portion through the bladder neck and that the

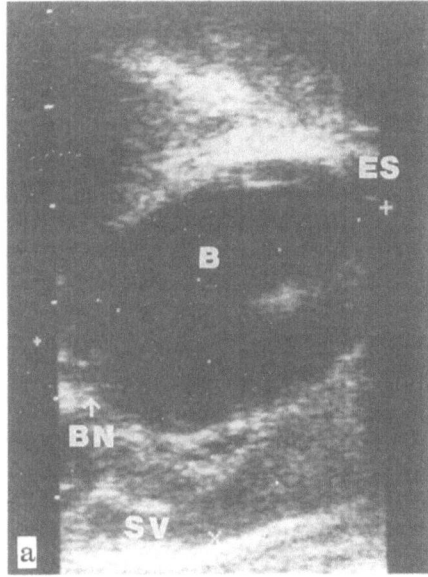

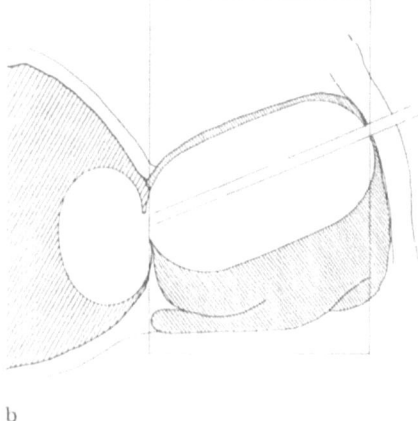

b

Fig. 13. a Midsaggital transverse transrectal ultrasound (TRUS) scan during dilatation with the ASI Uroplasty catheter. Note how the prostate is being dilated in its entire length from the bladder neck (*BN*) to the external sphincter. (*BN*, bladder neck, *B* balloon; *ES*, external sphincter; *SV*, seminal vesical). **b** TRUS of area shown in **a** is within the *solid line square*

remaining tissue was being compressed distally around the catheter (Fig. 15, 16). It seems that at the apex of the prostate the tissue was not stretched around the balloon but was buckled or compressed against the membranous urethra. On digital rectal examination the catheter's palpating nodule or positioning collar seemed to remain static in its position with respect to the urethra and rectal palpating finger and

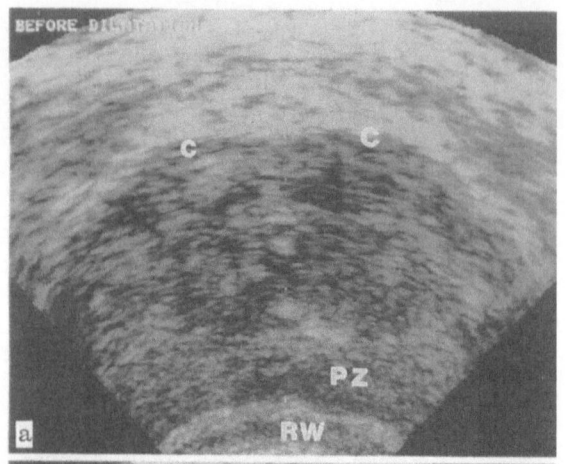

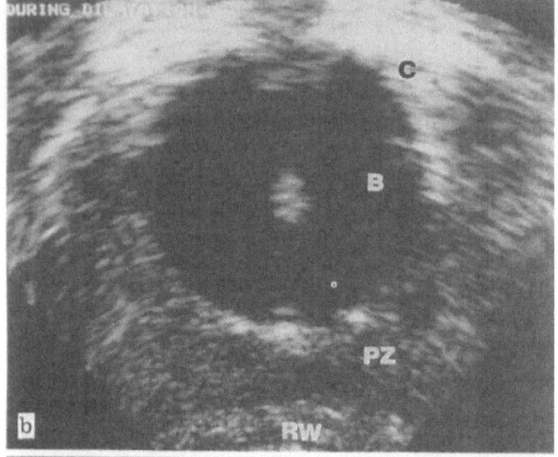

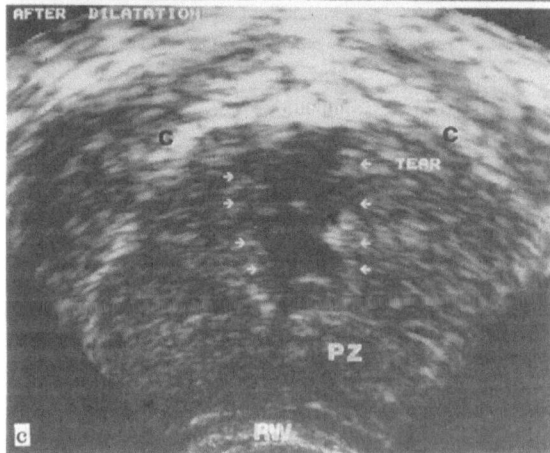

became more difficult to feel within this bulging tissue. In this study, each single-length balloon was removed and immediately replaced by a sized-to-fit system which was seen to "encapsulate" and stretch the prostate along its entire length (Fig. 12, 13). This basic difference in dilatation effect may help to explain the differences in clinical experience between different balloon systems.

Some Clinical Results

At the time of this writing there are considerable numbers of unpublished scientific presentations regarding balloon dilatation of the prostate. The few peer-reviewed published series that are available (Castaneda et al. 1987; Daughtry et al. 1990; Goldenberg et al. 1990; Marks 1992; Wasserman et al. 1990) are diverse in their criteria of patient selection, treatment methods, definitions of response, and duration of follow-up. Despite this, however, there is a growing common experience that suggests a degree of benefit from balloon dilatation, particularly in a subgroup of patients.

The four most mature series report a significant subjective improvement in 66%–85% of patients at 12 months (Castaneda et al. 1987; Daughtry et al. 1990; Goldenberg et al. 1990; Wasserman et al. 1990). Marks (1992) and Reddy et al. (1991) selected subgroups of patients with ideal characteristics and found that 88%–92% were satisfied with the outcome of dilatation after 12 months. In a longer follow-up study, Wasserman et al. report a mean symptom score improvement of 41% after 36 months (Wasserman et al. 1990). Other more anecdotal series (such as in unpublished presentations) fall into the same subjective improvement range. In a prospective randomized trial of balloon dilatation vs transurethral prostatectomy (Kreder et al. 1991) (n=52), Kreder and associates found a statistically significant decrease in symptom score from preoperative levels in both groups at 1 year follow-up (TURP 13.6 to 6.0; balloon 14.1 to 8.1). There was no significant difference between the groups with respect to symptoms. In fact, an equal percentage of patients (76%) in each arm considered themselves improved by their procedure.

The early subjective response rates must be considered in light of both the recognized placebo effect (as much as 40% in the management of benign prostatic hyperplasia) and the natural variability of obstructive and irritative voiding

---

Fig. 14. a Transverse transrectal ultrasound (TRUS) scan at the mid-prostate level prior to dilatation. Anterior-posterior distance is 2.4 cm; peripheral zone (*PZ*) is 0.6 cm; *RW*, rectal wall; *C* anterior capsule. **b** Transverse TRUS scan at same level during dilatation with the Uroplasty balloon system. Note that the capsular stretching and compression of the adenoma occurs primarily in the anterior fibromuscular stroma, with minimal distortion of peripheral zone tissue; *B* balloon; *C* capsule; *PZ*, peripheral zone; *RW*, rectal wall. **c** Transverse TRUS scan at same level following dilatation. Note the midline tear (*arrows*) extending from urethra to capsule; *RW*, rectal wall; PZ, peripheral zone

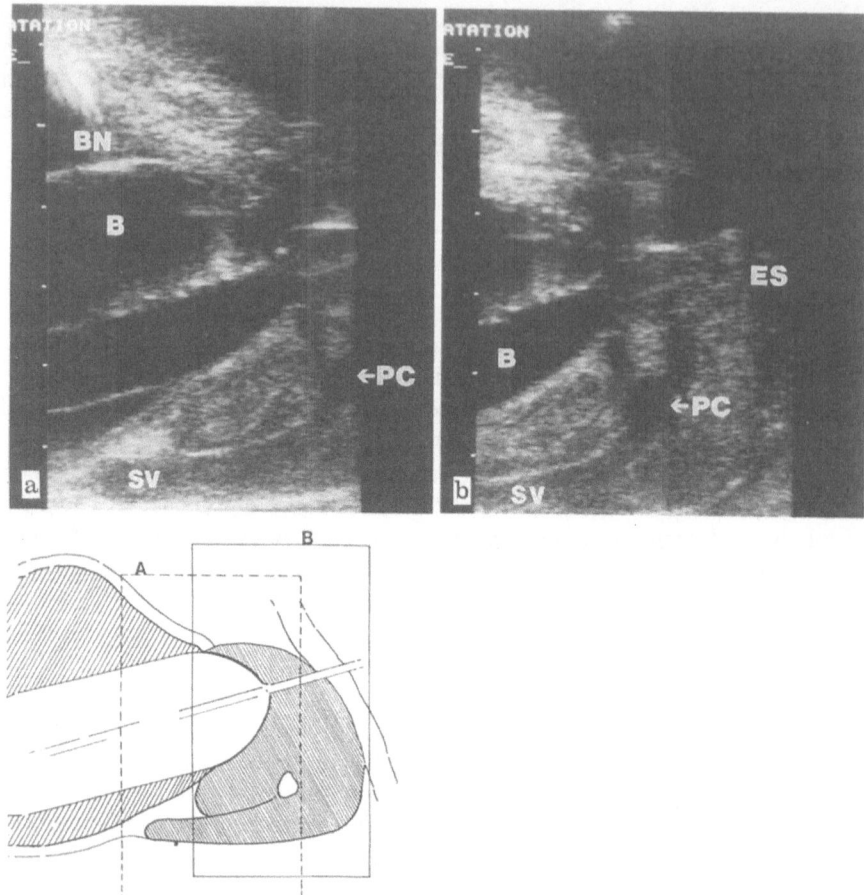

Fig. 15. a, b Midsaggital transverse transrectal ultrasound (TRUS) scans during dilatation with the Microvasive Dowd II catheter in the same patient as in Fig. 12. Note how the prostate is being dilated only in its proximal portion through the bladder neck. The prostatic cyst is a convenient reference point in these scans. (*PC*, prostate cyst; *BN*, bladder neck; *B*, balloon; *ES*, external sphincter; *SV*, seminal vesical). **c** TRUS of dashed line square (including prostatovesical junction) shown in **a**; TRUS of solid line square (including apical prostate and sphincter) shown in **b**

symptoms during the early course of this disease. The persistence of positive results from balloon dilatation beyond 12 months of follow-up indicates a true beneficial response to treatment rather than placebo or natural history.

In my series, all 153 patients treated with the Uroplasty balloon dilatation system were unequivocally obstructed, as determined by symptomatology, endoscopy, and urodynamics. These patients tended to be quite young (mean and median age of 63 years, range 45–81 years), with relatively small prostates (median weight 20 g, range 9–50 g). The mean Boyarsky symptom score of the patients was 14.8 prior

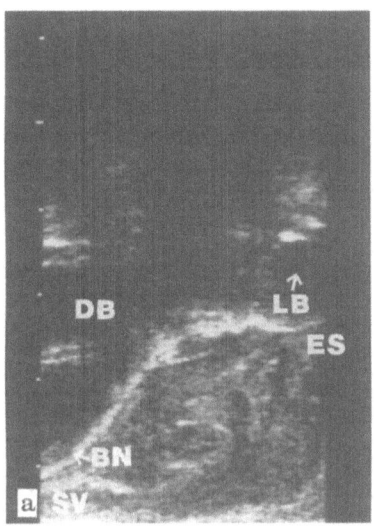 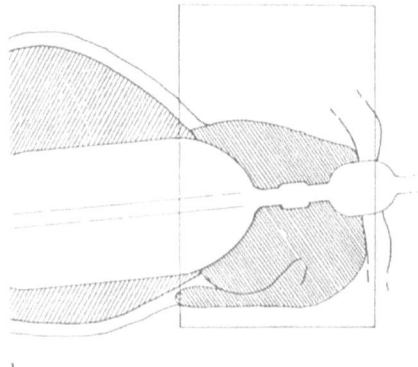

Fig. 16. a midsaggital transverse transrectal ultrasound (TRUS) scan during dilatation with the AMS Optilume catheter in the same patient as in Fig. 13. Note how the prostate is being dilated only in its proximal portion through the bladder neck. (*BN*, bladder neck; *DB*, dilating balloon; *LB*, locating balloon; *ES*, external sphincter; *SV*, seminal vesical). **b** TRUS of area shown in **a** is within the *solid line square*

to balloon dilatation and this decreased by 68% to a mean of 4.7 after 12 months and 5.8 (53% reduction) after 24 months of follow-up (Table 1).

Urodynamic evaluation included peak flow rate, mean flow rate, corrected flow rate (percentage of expected value for given voided volume, Siroky nomogram), postvoid residual, cystometrogram, and pressure-flow study. The peak flow rate increased from a pretreatment mean of 11.4 ml/s to 17.8 ml/s at 12 months (56% improvement) and 12.8 ml/s at 24 months (12% improvement). The corrected peak flow rates, which averaged 51% of expected value prior to treatment, increased to

Table 1. Summary of sympton scores (mean) and percent improvement at 6, 12, and 24 months follow-up

Symptoms	Preop: mean (*n*)	Follow-up (mean, (*n*), % improvement)		
		6 Months	12 Months	24 Months
Obstructive	10.5 (153)	3.1 (102)	2.6 (72)	3.7 (12)
		47	74	55
Irritative	4.3 (153)	2.1 (102)	2.1 (72)	2.1 (12)
		68	53	41
Total	14.8 (153)	5.2 (102)	4.7 (72)	5.8 (12)
		62	68	53

Table 2. Percent improvement in symptom scores at 6,12,18, and 24 months follow-up

Symptom score percent Improvement	Follow-up			
	6 Months ($n = 95$)	12 Months ($n = 69$)	18 Months ($n = 19$)	24 Months ($n = 12$)
>50	75 (79%)	58 (84%)	16 (84%)	7 (59%)
25–50	6 (6.3%)	7 (10%)	1 (5.3%)	4 (33%)
0–25	6 (6.3%)	3 (4.5%)	1 (5.3%)	1 (8%)
<0	8 (8.4%)	1 (1.5%)	1 (1.3%)	0 (0%)

75% of expected value at 12 months and returned to near baseline, 57%, at 24 months.

To date, 69 of our 153 patients have reached their 12 month evaluation. In this group 58 (84%) have had an excellent (greater than 50%) improvement in their symptom scores (Table 2). After 24 months, 11 of 12 patients remained satisfied with their treatment. (This statistic should be considered the "bottom line" since the ultimate determinant of success is the "happy patient.") When we look at the more objective evaluation of peak flow rate, only 40% have shown a comparable improvement at 12 months, while 22.5% actually had a deterioration in their Q_{max} (Table 3). Residual urine volumes have decreased but not with statistical significance. The discrepancies between subjective and objective response parameters are well recognized in studying the various treatment methods of Benign Prostatic Hypertrophy (BPH). The reasons for these discrepancies remain unexplained.

Balloon dilatation is well tolerated. All patients who are normally potent and have antegrade ejaculation preoperatively remain so after balloon dilatation. (In over 8000 transcystoscopic balloon dilatations performed worldwide there is yet to be a report of retrograde ejaculation or incontinence). Postoperative bleeding tends to be a moderate problem easily controlled by catheterization. Almost all patients have some bleeding around the Foley if an adequate tear is achieved with

Table 3. Percent improvement in peak flow rate, Q_{max} at 6,12,18, and 24 months follow-up

Q_{max} improvement (%)	Follow-up			
	6 Months ($n = 57$)	12 Months ($n = 40$)	18 Months ($n = 8$)	24 Months ($n = 5$)
>50	24 (42%)	16 (40%)	2 (25%)	0 (0%)
25–50	13 (23%)	6 (15%)	0 (0%)	1 (20%)
0–25	6 (10.5%)	9 (22.5%)	3 (37.5%)	2 (40%)
<0	14 (24.5%)	9 (22.5%)	3 (37.5%)	2 (40%)

the dilatation. Bladder irrigations may be discontinued within 6–8 h but the Foley catheter should be left indwelling for at least 48 h. In my early experience, when the catheter was removed after 24 h, two patients went into postoperative retention. This may have been due to clots or to edema. Since leaving the catheter in place for 48 h no patient has run into this problem.

Patients should be warned not to expect instant improvement after removal of the catheter. Voiding symptoms often persist for several weeks. Patients who exhibit a good response for the first 3 months continue to do well following balloon dilatation. Most failures present within the first 3 months after treatment.

Concluding Remarks

There is yet much to be learned about the mechanics of prostatic balloon dilatation. A multitude of equipment choices are on the market at this time including single length and sized-to-fit balloons, 75 F, 90 F, or 105 F diameters, locating buttons, and positioning balloons. I do not believe, however, that all types of balloon systems produce the same dilating effect on the full length of the prostate and prostate capsule. Intraoperative TRUS shows how a properly positioned sized-to-fit balloon achieves a full length compression of the gland and stretch of the capsule. In contrast, a single length balloon dilates and stretches the bladder neck but only displaces tissue at the apical portion of the gland (Fig. 12, 13, 15, 16). I believe that the dilatation of the apical portion of the prostate is more important than dilatation of the bladder neck. I make this point because of a group of patients who were treated for primary bladder neck hyperplasia with minimal lateral lobe enlargement (Goldenberg and Perez-Marerro 1990) and have responded well to dilatation without endoscopic or radiologic disruption of the bladder neck. Their resolution of symptoms can be explained by capsular distention causing an alteration or disruption of neuroreceptor activity. When using the single length balloon system one should consider repositioning the catheter (several times if necessary) to ensure a full length dilatation.

Careful patient evaluation, selection, and proper technique are undoubtedly the most important factors in ensuring a good response to balloon dilatation. An appropriate candidate is the young man (less than 65 years of age) with an "executive" prostate. That is, his prostate is small, he is sexually active with an interest in maintaining antegrade ejaculation, and he has clear cut symptomatic, urodynamic, and cystoscopic evidence of obstruction. Because of the nature of his lifestyle a 2–3 day recuperative time from balloon dilatation is much more acceptable than the several weeks required following prostatectomy or transurethral incisions. He may have failed, or have a contraindication to, pharmacologic therapy such as α-blockers. The ideal patient characteristics will be further defined as more studies come to maturation.

There are certain patient qualities that generally predict failure of balloon dilatation. These include an obstructing median lobe, multiple prostatic calculi, urethral stricture disease, chronic prostatitis, large gland (greater than 40–50 g), unstable bladder, or high residual urines (greater than 50% of bladder capacity). Ongoing studies using pressure-flow nomograms may make it easier to identify these poor candidates.

In summary, balloon dilatation is one of an expanding group of alternatives that are arriving in the marketplace for the treatment of benign prostatic hyperplasia. It has shown beneficial effects in treating bladder outlet obstruction in properly selected patients, but it will not replace an appropriate transurethral resection of the prostate any more than a transurethral resection would substitute for open enucleation when this procedure is indicated. Patients tolerate balloon dilatation extremely well, are usually able to return to work within 2–3 days, and maintain normal ejaculation and continence. Balloon dilatation may be repeated and does not preclude going on to a transurethral resection in the patient who has not shown an improvement.

Many questions regarding balloon selection, techniques, patient evaluation, patient selection, and duration of response remain to be answered before the definitive position of prostatic balloon dilatation is established in the urological armamentarium.

Acknowledgement. Special thanks to Dr. Dan Murray for his assistance with the transrectal ultrasound scans.

References

Aalkjaer V (1965) Transurethral resection/prostatectomy versus dilatation treatment in hypertrophy of the prostate. Urol Int 20:17–22

Backman K-A (1963) Dilatation of the prostate according to Deisting. Acta Chir Scand 126:266–274

Burhenne HJ, Chisholm RJ, Quenville NF (1984) Prostatic hyperplasia: radiological intervention. Radiology 152:655–657

Caine M (1986) The present role of alpha-adrenergic blockers in the treatment of benign prostatic hypertrophy. J Urol 136:1–4

Castaneda F, Reddy PK, Wasserman N et al. (1987) Benign prostatic hypertrophy: retrograde transurethral dilation of the prostatic urethra in humans. Radiology 163:649

Daughtry JD, Rodan BA, Bean WJ (1990) Balloon dilation of prostatic urethra. Urology 36:203–209

Deisting, W (1956) Transurethral dilatation of the prostate: a new method in the treatment of prostatic hypertrophy. Urol Int 2: 158–171

Goldenberg SL, Perez-Marerro RA (1992) Mechanism of prostatic balloon dilatation In: Castaneda F (ed) Therapeutic alternatives in the management of benign prostatic hyperplasia (Thieme Medical Publishers New York, 1992. pp. 77–82

Goldenberg SL, Perez-Marerro RA, Lee LM, Emerson L (1990) Endoscopic balloon dilatation of the prostate: early experience. J Urol 144:83–88

Hollingsworth E (1910) Dilatation of the prostatic urethra for the relief of symptoms of prostatic enlargement. Ann Surg 51:597–599

Klein LA, Leeming B (1988) Balloon dilatation for prostatic obstruction: long term follow-up. Presented at the 83rd annual meeting of the AUA, Boston, abstract 444

Kreder KJ, Donatucci CF, Crawford ED, Donohue RE, Whitesel J, Yakely R, Berger N (1991) Balloon dilation of the prostate versus transurethral resection: a continuing prospective, randomized clinical trial. Annual meeting of the AUA, Washington DC

Lepor H (1989) Nonoperative management of benign prostatic hyperplasia. J Urol 141:1283–1289

Marks LS (1992) Value of balloon dilation in treatment of youthful patients with prostatism. Urology 39:31–38

Moseley WG (1992) Balloon dilatation of prostate: keys to sustained favorable results. Urology 39:314–318

Quinn SF, Dryer R, Smathers R, Glass T, Wright E, Roberts C, Burke J, Argenbright J (1985) Balloon dilatation of the prostatic urethra. Radiology 157:57–58

Reddy PK, Wasserman N, Castaneda F, Castaneda-Zuniga WR (1987) Transurethral balloon dilatation of the prostate for prostatism: preliminary report of nonsurgical technique. J Endourol 1:269–273

Reddy PK, Wasserman N, Castaneda F, Castaneda-Zuniga WR (1988) Balloon dilatation of the prostate for treatment of benign hyperplasia. Urol Clin North Am 15:529–535

Reddy PK, Wasserman NF, Berg PA, Zhang G, Kapoor DA (1991) Patient selection predicts outcome following balloon dilation of the prostate. Annual meeting of the American Urological Association, Toronto, abstract #597

Sandberg I, Sandstrom B (1967) Dilatation according to Deisting for prostatic hyperplasia. Scand J Urol Nephrol 1:225–226

Wasserman NF, Reddy PK, Zhang G, Berg PA (1990) Experimental treatment of benign prostatic hyperplasia with transurethral balloon dilation of the prostate: preliminary study in 73 humans. Radiology 177: 485–494

Prostate Urethral Prostheses

S.A.Kaplan

Introduction

Of all the new alternative therapeutic measures under investigation for the management of symptomatic prostatism, the one which makes the greatest intuitive sense to urologists is prostate stents. The notion of implanting a device, transurethrally, to "open up" the prostatic urethra is inherent to basic urologic management of prostate obstruction. Therefore, it is not surprising that there has been considerable enthusiasm, as well as early encouraging results, in the use of prostate endoprostheses.

This has been particularly true in elderly or debilitated patients with benign prostatic hyperplasia (BPH) who often have multiple contraindications to surgical removal of bladder outlet obstruction (Kaplan and Koo 1990). These patients are often destined to long-term indwelling bladder catheterization which is often accompanied by multiple sequelae including urinary tract infection and sepsis, uremia, and renal insufficiency. In addition, these patients require close monitoring and frequent catheter changes with attendant inconvenience to the patient and medical costs. The purpose of this chapter is to provide an up to date review of the use of endoprostheses in the prostatic urethra.

Endoprostheses in Medicine

Other specialties in medicine have applied this basic concept, that is, placement of a stent through a stenotic lumen, for the past two decades (Table 1). This is particularly true in the field of vascular surgery. In 1969, Dotter et al. reported on the use of a coilspring in the popliteal artery. More recently, there have been reports of successful stenting of coronary arteries, although stringent anticoagulation is necessary (Bucx et al. 1991). Self-expandable stents of stainless steel (Wallstent) were used in 26 iliac and 15 femoral-popliteal artery lesions of 31 patients to treat stenoses or occlusions. The indications were confined to complex lesions, including residual stenoses and dissections after percutaneous procedures or previous surgery in the iliac artery lesions, and long-segment (mean, 13.5 cm) occlusions with inadequate response to percutaneous recanalization in the femoropopliteal artery

Table 1. Role of endoprostheses in medicine

Vascular
Coronary
Peripheral (iliac, femoral, popliteal)
Renal artery
GI tract
Biliary
Urologic
Urethral strictures
Detrusor - external sphincter dyssynergia
Renal artery stenosis
Benign prostatic Hypertrophy

lesions. In the iliac artery group, after stent placement, 96% of the lesions were patent at a mean follow-up of 16 months while in the femoropopliteal artery group, in 11 patients, only six had patent stents at 7–26 months (Zollikofer et al. 1991). This is consistent with the work of others who have reported greater success in larger diameter vessels (Rousseau et al. 1987). Finally, the successful use of plastic biliary endoprostheses to relieve malignant obstructive jaundice in 80%–90% of the patients was recently reported (Foerster et al. 1991). The authors recommended that because of the comfort of a completely indwelling endoprosthesis, it should be offered to all palliatively treated tumor patients, and external-internal catheters should be reserved for the minority of patients who return with reoccluded endoprostheses.

Endoprostheses in Urology

There have been a host of endoprostheses proposed and investigated in the management of urologic disorders, including urethral strictures, detrusor-external sphincter dyssynergia, and renal artery stenosis. A multicenter European group (Ashken et al. 1991) reported on the use of the Wallstent in 71 patients with bulbar urethral strictures. Fifty patients had previous urethral dilatations, 68 optical urethrotomies. The stent was always placed distal to the external urethral sphincter. Subjectively, 68 of 71 patients were satisfied with the results. Flow rates improved from 6 ml/s to 18 ml/s at 8 months. Retrograde urethrography performed in 27 patients at least 3 months poststent insertion revealed patency of the urethra. At 12 months, 23 stents were covered with a smooth epithelium with no infection or encrustation noted. The most common side effects included perineal discomfort which occurred in most patients but was usually self-limiting. Persistent bleeding occurred in four patients during the first 3 months. Leekage of urine was noted in 28 patients at 3 months secondary to pooling in the urethra

Table 2. Prostatic urethral prostheses

Spirals
    Prostakath
    Urospiral

Self-Expandable stents
    Superalloy mesh (Wallstent)
    Stainless steel (Gianturco)

Balloon expandable
    Intraprostatic device (titanium)

On the horizon
    Intraurethral Stent
    Biodegradable (poly-L-lactide)
    Thermoexpandable (TiNi)

---

of serous discharge. In the majority of patients, this resolved. Parra, in 1991, reported on the successful use of a titanium stent in five patients with recurrent posterior urethral structures. Four have had unobstructed voiding with no evidence of incontinence. McInerney et al. (1991) reported on the use of the Wallstent in 22 patients with spinal cord injury and documented detrusor external sphincter dyssynergia. Fifteen patients achieved complete voiding after placement of one stent; three developed bladder neck obstruction after stenting, but in one of these patients this was resolved by incision of the bladder neck. Placement of the stent was predicted on the desire for future fertility; that is, placement of the stent distal to the verumontanum.

A stainless steel endoprosthesis was placed in 12 renal arteries of 11 patients; a total of 15 stents were placed (Wilms et al. 1991). Indications for placement were restenosis after dilation and insufficient result after dilation. Complications included a case of massive cholesterol embolization and a case of unexplained transient hematuria, proteinuria, and deterioration of renal function. At repeat angiography of seven renal arteries after stent placement, one was occluded and required thrombolysis and dilation. After a clinical follow-up of 6.7 months ±3.4 in ten patients treated for hypertension, three were cured, four were improved, and three were unchanged when blood pressure levels before stent placement were compared with those obtained after stent placement.

Prostate Spring

Prostakath

A prostatic stent or spiral was first described by Fabian in 1980. There have been many subsequent modifications including the Prostakath (Engineers & Doctors A/S,

124   S.A. Kaplan

Copenhagen, Denmark). The stent, which is composed of stainless steel, is coated with 24 carat gold which aids in preventing encrustation (Fig. 1). The outside diameter is 21F and comes in four lengths: 4.5, 5.5, 6.5, and 7.5 cm. The straight portion consisting of multiple spiral loops remains in the prostatic urethra with the most proximal portion extending through the bladder neck into the bladder. The distal portion consists of a 2 cm straight wire segment traversing the membranous urethra and two spiral loops in the bulbar urethra. It is important to note that the spiral *does not* become epithelialized.

The Prostakath can be placed either under direct vision or under ultrasound guidance. Vincente et al. (1991) reported on 49 patients (40 with BPH, seven with prostatic carcinoma and two patients with "sclerosis" of the bladder neck) who were followed up for 22 months after cystoscopic insertion. There was normal voiding in 74%, decreases postvoid residual in 88.5%, and flow rates between 6 and 12 ml/s in 60% of cases.

In a multicenter study from Finland, 75 patients underwent placement of the Prostakath (80% under ultrasound guidance). A good or excellent result was noted in 58% of patients, while eight remained in urinary retention. Three patients required removal of the Prostakath because of urinary tract infection (Ala-Opas et al. 1991). During 1 year, the stent was inserted in 26 men who were poor operative risks. The treatment was successful in 20 (77%), and all were able to void satisfactorily. Four of the 20 resumed sexual activity, which previously had been prevented by indwelling catheters. Two patients who had delayed prostatic surgery because of fear of impotence were able to empty their bladders properly and to remain sexually active. Three patients subsequently had surgery, two after anticoagulant therapy could be stopped and one after renal function improved. No difficulties caused by the stent were encountered during surgery. Four patients who had the stent in place for 12 months had no difficulties. In 16 of the 18 patients who had indwelling catheters and infected urine before insertion of the stent, sterilization of the urine was obtained after relatively short courses of antibiotic treatment. Short-term complications associated with the stent were incontinence or urinary retention. These were treated by repositioning the stent. Frequency of urination

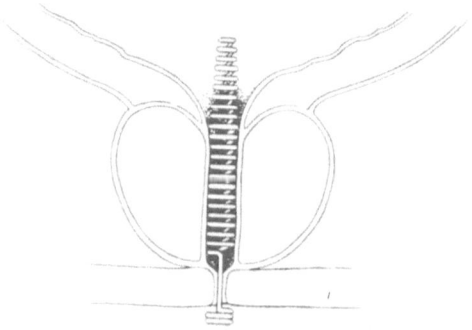

Fig. 1. The Protakath. Note the position of the spiral through the prostatic, membranous, and bulbar urethra

after insertion of the stent either disappeared spontaneously or was treated with anticholinergic drugs. In six patients, frequency was so severe that removal of the stent and insertion of an indwelling catheter were necessary. Slight to mild dysuria occurred immediately after surgery in all patients but eventually disappeared. Nordling et al. (1989) noted the successful use of ultrasound guidance for stent insertion: they reported that the in situ position was maintained at 3 months in 82% of patients. Some patients are more prone to experience stent migration because of either the length or the configuration of the prostatic urethra.

Porges Urospiral

Miller et al. (1991) recently reported that in 36 patients who underwent endoprostatic helicoplasty using a similar spiral, the Porges Urospiral, 67% had a successful outcome. A major predisposing factor for failure included patients with chronic retention. In addition, eight patients had incontinence. In a Turkish study, 18 patients were all able to void after stent insertion. However, 44% had persistent urinary tract infection and upward migration of the stent in 55% of cases (Karaoglan et al. 1991).

Self-Expandable Stents

Wallstent

The UroLume Wallstent (American Medical Systems) is a biomedical superalloy prosthesis woven in a tubular mesh and produced in various diameters and lengths (Fig. 2). It is stable when expanded and will not suffer elastic recoil. It is preloaded in a special delivery system that allows direct visualization of the prosthesis and the urethra throughout the entire insertion procedure. As the UroLume is deployed from the delivery system, it expands to a diameter of 14 mm. The elastic properties and radial force of the prosthesis allow it to remain in place and prevent migration.

The stent can be placed under spinal, caudal or local anaesthesia with a prostate block and IV sedation. In our experience, a saddle block has been particularly

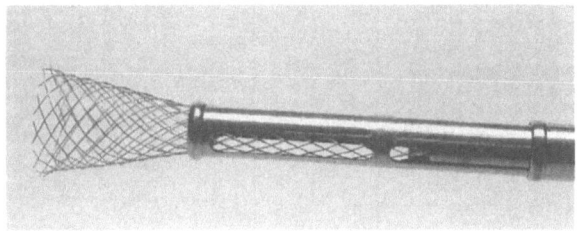

Fig. 2. Self-expanding stent (Wallstent) composed of a superalloy mesh

effective with minimal patient discomfort or morbidity. The length of the prostatic urethra is calibrated using either a standard ureter stent or a calibration catheter. A deployment tool (Fig. 1) is used to place the stent (2 or 3 cm in length) under direct vision (Fig. 3). In patients with longer prostatic urethras, overlapping stents can be used. This device contains the stent in a compressed state and is 21 F in diameter. As the stent is released, it expands to its full diameter and length. In our own experience and that of others, it has been determined that one of the keys to successful placement is that no portion of the stent protrude through the bladder neck into the bladder or distally beyond the verumontanum.

Chapple et al. (1990) reported their preliminary experience using the Wallstent in 12 patients with prostatic outflow obstruction. All were in a high risk group for surgery and 11 were treated successfully, with a follow-up of 1–11 months (median 9). The majority of patients (11 of 12) were satisfied with the procedure, which provided a quick, safe, and effective alternative to conventional surgical treatment. In this series, the stent was delivered using combined ultrasound and endoscopic control under local anaesthesia. The procedure was well tolerated, the stent becoming covered with epithelium by 6–8 months following insertion, yet allowing easy removal within the first 4–6 weeks should the need arise.

In that series, mean flow rate improved to 13.4 ± 4.7 ml/s. All patients had post-operative urgency which usually resolved within 4–6 weeks. However, in one patient, these symptoms persisted consistent with de novo detrusor instability.

The same group has updated their experience in 54 patients. The majority demonstrated marked objective and subjective improvement, while five stents required removal (Milroy et al. 1991). Harrison and De Souza (1990) reported a similar experience in 30 patients with outflow obstruction. Most had retention of urine and were unfit for conventional surgery. The prostatic stent was readily inserted under local anaesthesia and successfully relieved obstruction in 80% of patients with acute retention.

Finally, McLoughlin et al. (1990) reported that all 19 patients in urinary retention were able to void spontaneously after placement of the Wallstent. Similarly, a high percentage of patients reported postoperative urgency (79%) which resolved within 8 weeks. In a subsequent study, the same group reported that in 21 patients, endoprostheses were placed under fluoroscopic guidance. The procedure was technically successful in all patients, although in one a second stent was required 2

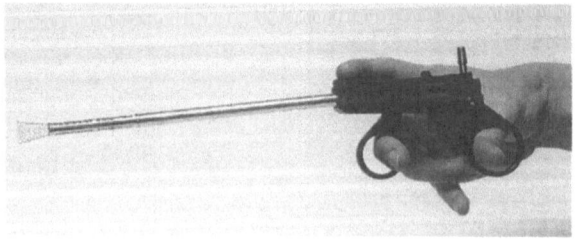

Fig. 3. Delivery tool. The stent is positioned at the bladder neck and distally to the verumontanum

months later (Adam et al. 1990). One patient developed a urethral stricture in the 12–16 month follow up-period. One patient with epididymoorchitis and one with septicemia after stenting were treated successfully with antibiotics.

In the United States, Oesterling, in 1991, reported on the use of the Wallstent in a different population, those with moderate symptoms yet relatively healthy. In 24 men (ages 62–77), symptoms scores decreased from 13.1 to 4.8. Urinary flow rates increased from 9.6 ml/s to 20.1 ml/s. Postvoid residual volume decreased from 107 ± 74 ml to 32 ± 14 ml. There were no cases of infection, encrustation, erosion, or migration. He similarly noted that the majority of patients experience postoperative urgency which resolves overtime. There is a current, ongoing, multicenter trial to investigate the use of the Wallstent in patients with symptomatic prostatism.

Gianturco Stent

A self-expanding metal stent, the Gianturco stent, has been recently investigated in the prostatic urethras of dogs (Dobben et al. 1991). The stent differs from the Wallstent in that it is stainless steel, has greater spacing between each of the interstices, is inserted with a stent pusher, and is 1.5 cm in diameter. There was no epithelial overgrowth and marked infiltration of lymphoid cells. There are currently no data available on its efficacy in humans.

Balloon Expandable Stents

Titanium Intraprostatic Stent

Titanium possesses excellent biocompatibility with a long history of safety as a biomaterial for both dental and orthopedic implants. It is particularly useful where stresses are moderate to low and where the implant is intended for long-term use. The intraprostatic stent, when expanded, is 11 mm in diameter and is available in lengths ranging from 12 to 65 mm in 4 mm increments (Fig. 4). The stent is placed cystoscopically under local anesthesia and sedation. As with the Wallstent, a calibration catheter is inserted cystoscopically and the length of the prostatic urethra from the bladder neck to the external urethral sphincter is measured under direct vision. The elongated stent is mounted on an insertion catheter which can be adapted to a special urethroscopic sheath (Fig. 5). The expansion of the stent in the prostatic urethra is performed by inflating the balloon on the insertion catheter to 130 psi (or 9 atm) for 30 s (Fig. 6). The position of the stent can be confirmed either cystoscopically or by ultrasound (Fig. 7). Adjustment of the position of the stent can be performed using grasping forceps through the cystoscope.

In a series from England, Kirby et al. (1991) noted that 28/32 patients in acute urinary retention were able to void satisfactory after placement of the intraprostatic stent. Asymptomatic urinary tract infections were noted in eight patients. In a more recent update of their data, 36/42 patients in retention were able to void spontaneously with a mean peak flow rate of 10.5 ml/s.

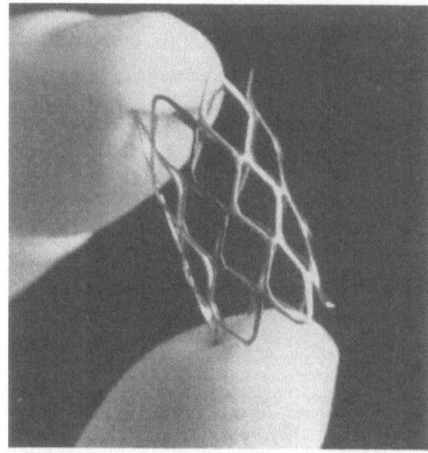

Fig. 4. Titanium stent

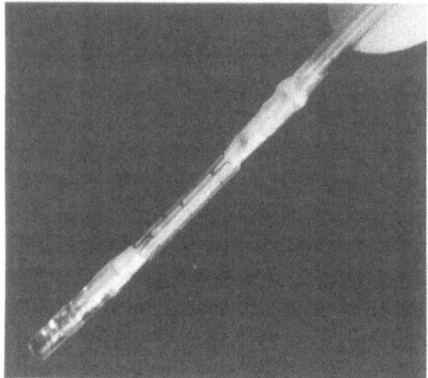

Fig. 5. Stent positioned on a specially designed inflation catheter

Recently, a multicenter, cooperative study representing the initial United States experience using the intraprostatic stent was conducted 44 patients (ages 60-93). All patients had a symptom score analysis and measurement of uroflow as part of their initial workup (Kaplan et al. 1992). Patients were seen at 1, 3, 6, and 12 months after stent insertion (mean follow-up=7 months). Of the 44 patients, 20 presented in urinary retention. The type of anesthesia included three general, 17 spinal or epidural, ten intravenous sedation, and 14 with intraurethral xylocaine only.

All patients were able to void spontaneously within 36 h after stent insertion. Symptoms scores decreased from 16 to 4, 7, 5 and 5 at 1, 3, 6 and 12 months, respectively. Peak uroflow increased from 7 ml/s to 13, 11, 11 and 13 ml/s at 1, 3, 6 and 12 months, respectively.

Of the initial 44 patients, five died from their underlying disorder (all voiding satisfactorily with the stent in place) and 17 underwent uneventful stent removal (ten technical failures and seven treatment failures). Technical failures were

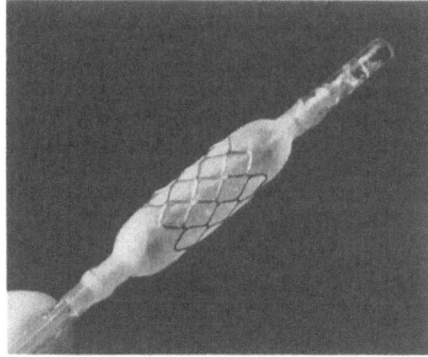

Fig. 6. The stent expanding to 33 F in diameter

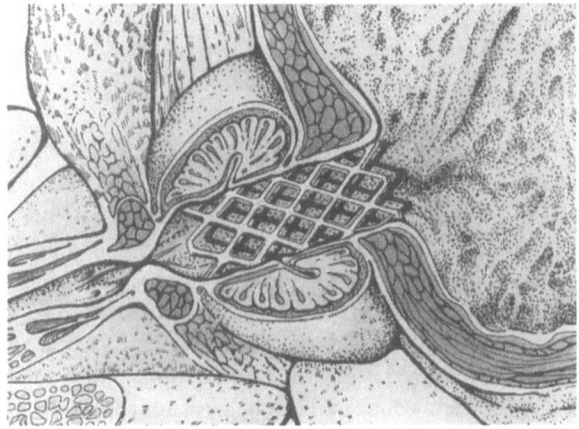

Fig. 7. The stent in proper position within the prostatic urethra

secondary to either inaccurate positioning or improper stent sizing. Of the 34 patients with proper placement of the stent, 29 (85%) had improvement of both symptom scores and uroflow. Transient hematuria was noted in 41 patients (93%) and usually resolved within 48 h.

On the Horizon

Intraurethral Catheter

Researchers in Israel have developed an intraurethral catheter as an alternative to long-term indwelling catheters. Nissenkorn and Lang (1991) placed 83 intraurethral catheters (IUC) in 65 patients between 1988 and 1990. All insertions were done under local anesthesia and in an outpatient setting. The IUC was left in place from 1 to 61 weeks (mean 19.4 weeks). All patients were able to void freely, were continent, and had no residual urine. In three patients there were unresolved urinary tract infections requiring removal of the IUC. In addition, patients who were sexually active prior to catheter placement were able to continue normal ejaculations with the IUC in place.

Biodegradable Stents

The advantages of a biodegradable stent is that there is no need for removal of the implanted material. A biodegradable spiral stent composed of poly-L-lactide (PLLA) with a length of 15 mm and diameter of 0.7 mm was implanted into 14 male rabbits. There were no calcifications noted and the stent was completely absorbed at 14 months. This early data suggests that this material may be a promising material for stents in the urinary tract (Kemppainen et al. 1991).

Thermoexpandable Stent

A stent made of an equiatomic intermetallic compound NiTinol (a titanium-nickel compound) has had early encouraging results in eight patients. The stent has the ability to change from one configuration to another at different temperatures. A NiTinol thread of 0.85 mm diameter is mounted on an insertion catheter as a coil with a diameter of 21 F. Flushing the catheter with 45°C water makes the coil expand to 35 F and the insertion catheter can then be removed. If the stent requires removal, the coil can be irrigated with 15°C which softens the metal allowing the coil to be removed as a string. Of the initial eight patients, four had stent migration during the procedure while four have remained for a minimum of 6 months with satisfactory voiding (Nordling et al. 1991).

Conclusions

The use of stents to bridge the prostatic urethra has met with considerable enthusiasm. Based on initial results, it seems quite clear that this technology will have a lasting impact on how we treat some patients with BPH. In our experience, the optimal patient has been the frail elderly patient in urinary retention. Others have advocated endoprostheses, particularly the prostatic spiral, as "stress tests" to determine how patients will fare after definitive prostatectomy (McLoughlin and Williams 1990).

However, future prospects, particularly the use of biodegradable materials, should make the prostatic stent more potentially attractive to a greater segment of the BPH population. Future studies will help direct the urologist in selecting: (1) the appropriate clinical setting for use of the prostate stent and (2) what type of stent to use.

References

Adam A, Jager R, McLoughlin J, elDin A, Machan L, Williams G, Allison DJ (1990) Wallstent endoprostheses for the relief of prostatic urethral obstruction in high risk patients. Radiology 42(4):228-232

Ala-Opas M, Talja M, Hellstrom P, Tititinen J, Heikkinen, Nurmi M (1991) Prostakath - urospiral in urinary outflow obstruction. Presented at the Societé Internationale d'Urologie, Seville 1991 (abstract 622)

Ashken MH, Coulange C, Milroy EJG, Sarramon JP (1991) European experience with the urethral Wallstent for urethral structures. Eur Urol 19:181-185

Bucx JJ, deCheerder I, Beatt K, dvandenBrand M, Suryapranata H, deFeyter PJ, Serruys PW (1991) The importance of adequate anticoagulation to prevent early thrombosis after stenting of stenosed venous bypass grafts. Am Heart J 121(5):1389-1396

Chapple CR, Milroy EJ, Rickards D (1990) Permanently implanted urethral stent for prostatic obstruction in the unfit patient: preliminary report. Br J Urol 66(1):58-65

Dobben RL, Wright KC, Dolenz K, Wallace S, Gianturco C (1991) Prostatic urethra dilatation with the Gianturco self-expanding metallic stent: a feasibility study in cadaver specimens and dogs. Am J Roentgenol 156(4):757-761

Dotter CT, (1969)

Dotter CT, Buschmann RW, McKinney MK et al. (1983) Transluminal expandable nitinol coil stent grafting: preliminary report. Radiology 147:259-260

Fabian KW (1980) Der intraprostatische "partielle Katheter" (urologische Spirale). Urologe (A) 19:236-238

Foerster EC, Hoepffner N, Domschke W (1991) Bridging of benign choledochal stenoses by endoscopic retrograde implantation of mesh stents. Endoscopy 23(3):133-135

Harrison NW, DeSouza JV (1990) Prostatic stenting for outflow obstruction. Br J Urol 65(2):192-196

Kaplan SA, Koo HP (1990) Prostatic stents. Curr Techn Urol 3:1-8

Kaplan SA, Parra R, Merrill DC, Benson RC, Chiou RK, Fuselier HA, Montague DK, Mosely W (1992) The titanium prostatic urethral stent: the United States experience (in press)

Karaoglan U, Alkibay T, Tokucoglu H, Deniz H, Bozkirli I (1991) Urospiral in benign prostatic hyperplasia. Presented at the Societé Internationale d'Urologie, Seville 1991 (abstract 621)

Kemppainnen E, Riihela M, Pohjonen T, Tormala P, Talja M (1991) Biodegradable urethral stent: an experimental study. Presented at the Société Internationale d'Urologie, Seville 1991 (abstract 625)

Kirby R, Lui S, Eardley I, Miller P, Christmas T, Vale J (1991) The use of the ASI titanium intraprostatic stent in the treatment of acute urinary retention due to BPH. Presented at the Société Internationale d'Urologie, Seville 1991 (abstract 620)

McInerney PD, Vanner TF, Harris SAB, Stephenson TP (1991) Permanent urethral stents for detrusor sphincter dyssynergia. Br J Urol 67:291-294

McLoughlin J, Williams G (1990) Prostatic stents and balloon dilatation. Br J Hosp Med 43:422-426

McLoughlin J, Jager R, Abel PD, elDin A, Adam A, Williams G (1990) The use of prostatic stents in patients with urinary retention who are unfit for surgery. An interin report. Br J Urol 66(1):66-70

Miller RA, Birch BR, Parker CJ (1991) Endoprostatic helicoplasty: the porges urospiral. J Urol 145:397A

Milroy E, Chapple CR, Rickards D (1991) Permanently implanted prostate stent - the urolume wallstent. J Urol 145:268A

Nissenkorn I, Lang R (1991) The intraurethral catheter, an alternative to the indwelling catheter with negligible infectuous complications. Presented at the Société Internationale d'Urologie, Seville 1991 (abstract 624)

Nordling J, Holm HH, Klarskov P, Neilsen KK, Andersen JT (1989) The intraprostatic spiral: a new device for insertion with the patient under local anaesthesia and with ultrasonic guidance with 3 months of followup. J Urol 142:756-758

Nordling J, Harboe H, Jacobsen E (1991) A termoexpandable stent for the treatment of prostatic obstruction. Presented at the Société International d'Urologie, Seville 1991 (abstract 582)

Oesterling JE (1991) The obstructive prostate and the intraurethral stent. Contemp Urol 3(10):61-72

Parra RO (1991) Treatment of posterior urethral strictures with a titanium urethral stent. J Urol 146(4):997-1000

Rousseau H, Puel J, Mirkovitch V et al. (1987) Self expanding endovascular prosthesis: an experimental study. Radiology 164:709-714

Vincente J, Salvador J, Izquierdo F, Caparros J (1991) Long term follow up of patients with intraprostatic prostheses. Presented at the Société Internationale d'Urologie, Seville 1991 (abstract 617)

Wilms GE, Peene PT, Baert AL, Nevelsteen AA, Suy RM, Verhaeghe RH, Vermylen JG and Fagard RH (1991) Renal artery stent placement with the use of the Wallstent endoprosthesis. Radiology 179(2):457–462

Yachia D, Lask D, Rabinson S (1990) Self-retaining intraurethral stent: an alternative to long-term indwelling catheters or surgery in the treatment of prostatism. Am J Roentgenol 154(1):111–113

Zollikofer CL, Antonucci F, Pfyffer M, Redha F, Salomonowitz E, Stuckmann G, Largiader I, Marty A (1991) Arterial stent placement with use of the Wallstent: midterm results of clinical experience. Radiology 179(2):449–456

Prostatic Heat Treatments

A.P.Perlmutter

Introduction

One of the new treatment regimes available for symptomatic benign prostatic hyperplasia (BPH) involves heating the prostate. This rapidly evolving technique aims to provide relief to obstructed patients in an outpatient setting with minimal anesthesia. The term "hyperthermia" has become associated with the current trend for heat treatment of the prostate, but it has its origin in the treatment of malignant tissue. Indeed, the initial experience with transrectal microwave probes was gained in treating prostatic cancer. An applicator containing a microwave antenna was developed which could be placed into the rectum and aimed at the prostate. This energy delivery system allowed controlled heating of the prostate to specific temperatures within a confined space. The treatments for prostatic cancer were based on the observation that malignant tissue, but not normal tissue, was susceptible to temperatures of 42°–43.5°C. This temperature range has been adopted by some of the current devices to treat BPH, and the use of the term "hyperthermia" is thus restricted to define those treatments which developed directly from cancer therapy and which heat to <44°C. Hyperthermia treatments for BPH are delivered by microwave antennae placed in the rectum and do not cause tissue necrosis.

The development of devices to deliver energy from antennae placed on modified urethral catheters has resulted in the attainment of treatment temperatures in excess of 44.5°C. These antennae are localized on the portion of the catheter which is intraprostatic, and transurethral devices heat the prostate with the additional goal of attaining permanent tissue destruction. Treatment with devices which heat to greater than 44.5°C is referred to as "thermotherapy." The distinction is warranted since necrosis of normal tissue is achieved at the higher temperatures and thus different mechanisms may be responsible for clinical efficacy.

Over the past 10 years, a variety of both transrectal and transurethral antennae have been developed which deliver a multitude of radio frequencies to the prostate. Different devices heat the prostate to different temperatures for different periods of time, and the relative efficacy of hyperthermia vs thermotherapy is not established. There are no generally accepted treatment protocols which define optimal patient selection, treatment temperature, or treatment time, and the mechanisms responsible for the clinical effect are not completely known. Prostatic heat treatments are currently investigatory, and their role in treating symptomatic BPH is yet to be established.

Historical Background

Microwave Principles

Interest in heat treatments for medical therapy reportedly began as early as 2000 B.C. (Yerushalmi 1975), and the beneficial effects of heat in the treatment of neoplasm have been known since 1866 when Busch reported the regression of a sarcoma following a severe febrile episode. During the 1970s, investigation began into the heat sensitivity of tumor tissue. Although many methods are available for heating tissue, microwave energy is clinically useful because it can be easily generated in a controlled manner with small applicators and antennae. Microwaves are transverse electromagnetic waves with frequencies from 30 to 3000 MHz. The basic physical properties governing the development of clinical treatment devices are that these waves propagate in free space or in a medium and are reflected or scattered at interfaces of two media with different impedance. This electromagnetic radiation heats by inputting energy into biologic tissue by the displacement or drift of free charge, the polarization of atoms and molecules, and the orientational polarization of existing dipoles. Thus, the heating pattern obtained by the device depends on the distribution of energy in the target tissues resulting from the incident microwave field. This is determined by: (1) the intensity distribution within the generated field, (2) applicator size and shape, (3) frequency of operation, (4) size and shape of tissue contours, and (5) the electrical properties of the tissues being penetrated by the field (Paliwal and Shrivastava 1989). Lower frequency microwaves have greater tissue penetration due to a longer wavelength but require larger applicators. The initial transrectal applicators used for prostatic heating emitted 915 MHz.

The devices used for microwave heat treatments consist of a computer control workstation connected to the hardware which is placed in the patient, and all have certain similar major components. A power generator is responsible for the microwave emission and an impedance matching network allows efficient transfer of power from generator to the antenna. The devices have a thermometry system which allows temperatures to be measured during therapy. The production of thermosensors which are neither heated by nor perturb the energy flow pattern is an important part of sophisticated microwave technology (Katzir et al. 1989). The temperature sensors feedback to the temperature controller which regulates the power delivered to the antenna so that the treatment temperature can be maintained in a narrow range. Finally, each device has computer storage capacity to record treatment data. The attainment of uniform temperature profiles is complicated by the variation in prostate shape and size and the heterogeneity of tissue types and vascularity both within a single prostate and between different patients.

Animal Trials

Microwave delivery systems designed to heat prostatic tissue were first applied to a dog model. The goal of this research was to cause tissue ablation at temperatures beyond the hyperthermia range. Magin et al. (1980) treated eight dog prostates with 2450 MHz radiation to 60°C for 15 min using an open survival surgery technique which shielded adjacent tissues. Bilateral cutaneous ureterostomies were created to provide urinary diversion. One half of the animals were sacrificed at 1 week posttherapy, and although prostatic volume was unchanged, detailed examination revealed that the tissue was completely devitalized and mummified, consistent with coagulation necrosis. The remaining four dogs were sacrificed at 6 months and histopathologic examination revealed that the prostate was replaced by fibrous scar. Harada et al. (1985) developed a transurethral 2450 MHz probe and treated 20 dogs for 1 min at 50–100 watts. Peak temperatures were believed to be in excess of 50°C. Postoperative catheterization was not necessary, and post procedure urethrograms revealed an enlarged prostatic fossa. Extensive necrosis and hemorrhage was noted on pathologic examination immediately postprocedure, and at 14 days central necrosis of the prostate was evident and fibrous tissue was noted at the periphery of the heated area. These experiments established that microwave energy could be used for prostatic tissue ablation.

The histopathologic changes which occur in the canine prostate after heat treatment were studied as an adjunct to initiating human treatment trials. Lieb et al. (1986) examined the prostates of 20 male dogs after heat treatment with the 915 MHz water-cooled skirt antenna being developed for human trials. Treatments from 40°C to 47°C were performed in order to assess device safety and the tissue effect of treatment in the hyperthermia range (42°–44°C) and at temperatures slightly lower or higher. They found that six 90 min treatments at 42.5°C resulted in diffuse, mononuclear cell infiltration and edema, but no observable irreversible or severe damage. In contrast, treatment at 44.5°C for six 90 min treatments resulted in necrosis of the prostatic urethra, hemorrhage, and inflammatory infiltration. Interestingly, a 15 min treatment at 47°C caused no observable damage, and thus the combination of treatment time and temperature is the governing parameter. Treatment at 40°C was completely safe even for 10 continuous hours and no histopathologic changes were observable. These studies provide the basis for many principles currently used in the human trials, although the canine prostate has a much higher gland:stroma ratio than does the human and is not an exact model for BPH. Treatment in the hyperthermia range of 42°–44°C is considered to be safe and without the ability to permanently change normal tissue, and treatment in the thermotherapy range of >44.5°C causes necrosis and therefore permanent change. Therefore, treatment of patients with obstructive BPH in the hyperthermic range is based on the hypothesis that the adenoma will be selectively sensitive to heat or that the treatment will result in a beneficial change in the normal prostatic capsule or adjacent bladder neck fibers which is not evident on simple histologic examination by hematoxylin and eosin stains. Thermotherapy treatment is designed to cause necrosis of the periurethral prostatic tissue and permanent shrinkage of the obstructing adenoma by fibrotic replacement.

The Transrectal Hyperthermia Experience

Since the rectal cavity allows easy access to the prostate with minimal patient discomfort, an applicator which is placed in the rectum and allows microwave energy to be directed toward the prostate was developed for prostatic heating. The microwave applicator heats by energy absorption, and a generalized heating profile of such a transrectal applicator is shown in Fig. 1a. At short distance from the applicator the temperature is high, and this temperature exponentially falls due to a combination of the penetration properties of the microwaves and the cooling effect of efferent blood flow. In a transrectal treatment, this results in the highest temperature range being achieved in the rectal wall rather than the prostate. In order to shift the maximum temperature away from the rectal wall, transrectal applicators contain circulating surface coolant which acts by conduction to reduce the temperature of adjacent rectal mucosa which is in direct contact with the applicator. An idealized temperature vs distance curve for any device which cools by conduction is depicted in Fig. 1b. The summation of heating by energy absorption and cooling by conduction is shown in Fig. 1c. This combination of temperature profiles shifts the heating process into the prostatic tissue and protects the rectal mucosa from thermal damage. The transrectal applicators in clinical use combine heating by energy absorption with cooling by conduction.

Hyperthermia for Malignancy

The initial human experience using microwave energy to heat the prostate was not directed toward prostatic ablation, but rather was gained in treating prostatic cancer. This treatment was developed because of the observation that neoplastic cells were more sensitive to heat than normal cells and were destroyed by hyperthermic temperatures of 42°–44°C (Song 1978). The temperature of maximum differential effect is midway between 40°C, at which neither tumor cells nor normal tissue are affected, and 45°C at which both cell types become necrotic after 1 h of treatment. The mechanism underlying the phenomenon that tumor cells are intrinsically more sensitive to heat than normal cells and thus can be selectively destroyed by heat is in part due to the vascular properties of the tumor itself. The tumor is not able to dissipate heat as rapidly as normal tissue due to poor vascularity and the reduced ability of tumor vessels to vasodilate (Matsuda et al. 1989; Nishimura et al. 1989). Heat accumulation is thus preferential and tumoricidal. In addition, neoplastic cells may be intrinsically more sensitive to heat possibly because they are relatively hypoxic, those cells in S-phase are very heat sensitive, and the heating process itself may stimulate immune modulators which result in tumor destruction.

In 1982, Yerushalmi et al. described the treatment of 15 patients with carcinoma of the prostate with transrectal "localized deep microwave hyperthermia." Four patients with stage B or C disease were treated with hyperthermia alone, the remaining 11 receiving both hormonal manipulation and hyperthermia. They observed that the treatments were well tolerated, and many of the treated patients

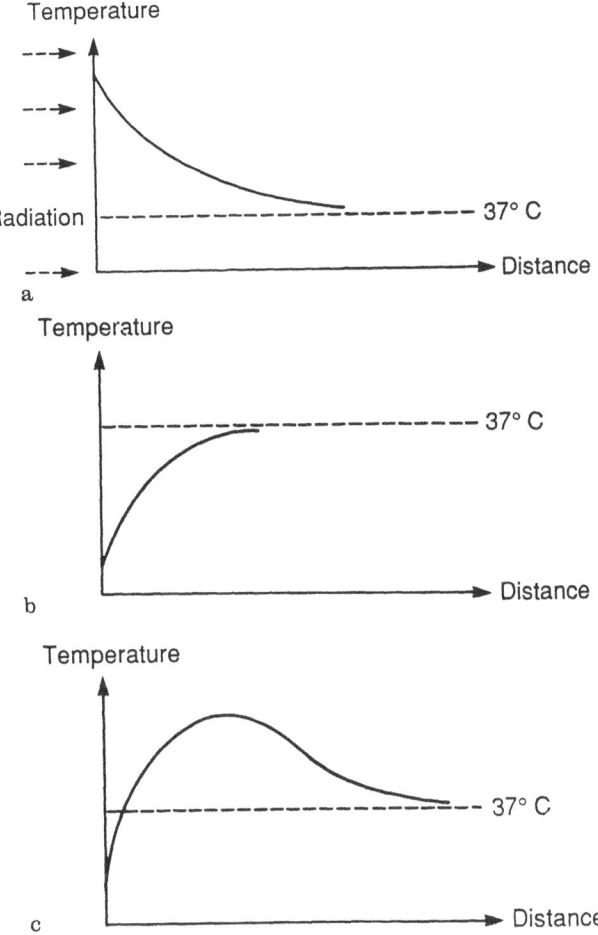

Fig. 1. a The generalized exponential decrease in temperature as distance increases from a heating source. **b** The generalized increase in temperature as distance increases from a cooling source in cooling by conduction. **c** The summation of **a** and **b** shows simultaneous heating by energy absorption and cooling by conduction

had a marked decrease in urinary frequency and dysuria. In addition, three patients who were in urinary retention were freed of their catheters after treatment with hyperthermia alone. Longer follow-up revealed that these patients maintained their improved voiding pattern at 6 months posttherapy, but that all had local progression and worsening of symptoms by 18 months (Servadio and Leib 1984). It was the observation that microwave hyperthermia improved the obstructive and irritative symptoms associated with prostatic outflow obstruction that led to the development of treatment devices and protocols for symptomatic BPH. Since the canine experience indicated that the normal prostatic tissue would not likely be permanently altered by hyperthermia, it was hoped that the prostatic adenoma would be analogous to carcinoma and possess similar selective heat sensitivity.

Initial Trials

Yerushalmi et al. (1985) published the first human trial using 2450 MHz transrectal microwave hyperthermia to treat a cohort of 29 poor operative risk patients with symptomatic, biopsy proven, BPH. Seven to 18 1 h treatments were given, and were well tolerated without evidence of rectal injury. Invasive thermometry verified peak temperatures of 42°–43°C in the prostate within 15 min of initiating treatment, and the rectal mucosa was cooled to below 32°C throughout treatment. Of the 11 patients in urinary retention prior to treatment, eight were freed of their catheters for 18 months of follow-up. Patients on average enjoyed a marked decrease in obstructive and irritative symptoms. In all patients who responded, the authors reported a decrease in prostatic size as determined by digital rectal examination.

The initial clinical experience with the Biodan Prostathermer (Biodan Medical Systems, Israel) was reported by Servadio et al. in 1986 who treated 32 patients for a total of 192 1 h sessions at 41°–43°C using a 915 MHz transrectal applicator incorporating rectal wall cooling. Treatment involved simultaneous transurethral catheterization with a catheter which incorporated a receiving antenna that facilitated the alignment of the microwave field and also incorporated a series of thermocouples that indicated intraprostatic temperatures. Newman and Knapp (1990) showed that the calculated maximal intraprostatic temperature bore a close relationship to the recorded maximal temperature, but that this bore no relationship to the power delivered by the rectal applicator. They also treated patients with carcinoma of the prostate and nonbacterial prostatitis, and this report sought to establish that the technique was safe and clinically feasible. They encountered two prostatorectal fistulae, both of which resolved after suprapubic drainage. This experience led to their 1987 report (Servadio et al. 1987) in which a cohort of 37 patients with severe symptomatic BPH who were poor surgical candidates were studied. They found that six to ten single hour sessions were required for clinical efficacy in the group of 29 treated patients; 13 of these patients were in urinary retention, and eight remained catheter-free at up to 24 months. The 16 patients with severe voiding symptoms had increased flow rates, a decrement in symptoms and postvoid residual urine volume, and a decrease in prostatic size from 24 to 20 ml. Eight patients were followed as controls and showed no improvement.

Optimization of Treatment Schedule and Patient Selection

In the same year and using the same device, Lindner et al. (1987) treated six patients in urinary retention from 1 to 6 months (mean 2.8) who had failed voiding trials on phenoxybenzamine. In developing a protocol for the number and duration of treatments, they used the thermal equivalent dose (TED) calculation to standardize the time-temperature relationship (Sapareto and Dewy 1984). This thermodynamic mathematical summation of temperature and time allowed Lindner et al. to compare different treatment regimes and establish six 1 h sessions as their standard protocol. They also investigated the relationship between the treatment temperature and the distance from the microwave applicator and determined that peak temperature is reached 15–20 mm from the rectal wall. Their calculations allow the prediction that temperature falls approximately 1°C for each 10 mm beyond the peak temperature zone. Five of the six patients were voiding at 6 months follow-up, with only one requiring continued α-blockade. Posttreatment peak flow rate reported for the five voiding patients was 20.4 ml/s, and digital rectal examination demonstrated a smaller prostate gland. An interesting aspect of this study is that none of the patients was able to void after treatment with α-blockade alone. Some authors (Watson et al. 1991) have speculated that the mechanism of hyperthermia action may be to reduce α-receptor mediated prostatic tone (Caine et al. 1978). If this were the case, successful treatment with α-blockade would be expected in a patient likely to benefit from hyperthermia, the opposite of the Lindner et al. (1987) experience.

Lindner et al. (1990a) further investigated the variables of treatment schedule and the use of cyproterone acetate (CPA) in the treatment of 72 men in urinary retention due to BPH who required a catheter after failing voiding trials on phenoxy-benzamine. They found five of 12 patients (41%) receiving three to five treatments for 1 h at 42°C were freed of their catheter compared to 13 of 26 (50%) patients receiving six to ten treatments. When concomitant CPA was given, four of 15 (27%) voided after three to five treatments and 14 of 19 (74%) voided after six to ten treatments. The difficulty encountered in delivering the proper thermal equivalent dose was noted by the fact that the majority of the 20 patients who were excluded because of infringement of protocol were so excluded because of discrepancies in thermal dose calculations. Complications, which resulted in four hospitalizations, included ten patients with fevers >38°C, rectal pain in 12, diarrhea in three, and hematuria in 11. They concluded that treatment with six to ten sessions is warranted, and that CPA is a useful adjunct in treating BPH.

The impact of CPA on hyperthermia efficacy was described by Lieb et al. (1991a,b). Whereas the pre- and 1 month posttreatment ultrasound determined prostatic volumes remained unchanged for those 55 patients treated by hyperthermia alone, there was a decrease from 83 ml to 67 ml for those treated simultaneously with hyperthermia and CPA. This effect was much less pronounced in the subgroup under 68 years of age. In a hyperthermia-treated subgroup which did not receive CPA, prostatic size increased slightly. This argues the better response reported above for large glands was the result of the CPA and not the hyperthermia. It is also possible that the CPA acts synergistically with the hyperthermia, resulting in an effect that would not be seen with CPA alone. These studies were also the first to use ultrasound determined volumes instead of digital exam approximation of prostatic size. The observations reported in this paper suggest that the previous digital rectal examinations of the hyperthermia-treated prostate gland, which found a reduction in volume, may not be correct, and that in fact hyperthermia alone has little effect on prostatic volume.

In an attempt to identify subgroups of patients more likely to have a positive response to treatment, Servadio et al. (1989) undertook a detailed analysis of 140 patients treated with the Prostathermer for obstructive BPH. The cohort as a whole had only a very small increase in peak flow rate from 10.1 ml to 12.8 ml/s and 11.9 ml/s at 1 and 6 months posttreatment, respectively. When the group was stratified by age (greater or less than 70 years old) and prostate size (greater or less than 85 ml), they found that those patients under 70 years old with prostates >85 ml had the best response. This group had a flow rate increase from 9.75 ml/s to 13.8 ml/s at 6 months, a 41% increase in flow. The second best performing group were those patients older than 70 with prostates >85 ml. The smallest response was observed in the group less than 70 years old with prostates <85 ml. Since CPA was also used in this study, the possible compounding effect of this anti-androgen makes it impossible to generalize the observation that larger prostates in younger patients responded most favorably.

Duration of Hyperthermia Effect

The duration of treatment effect was reported by Servadio et al. (1990) who followed 124 patients who were treated for symptomatic BPH for 1 year. This study contained a number of subgroups and demonstrated in controlled fashion that at least six treatments were necessary and that hourly treatment sessions at 41°–43°C were more efficacious than treatment at 39°–41°C. Thus, the threshold temperature at which the hyperthermia effect occurs is about 41°C. Improvement in objective parameters was most pronounced in those presenting with the most severe obstructive symptoms, and residual urine was effected to a greater amount than flow rate. They found 51% of patients had sustained improvement at 1 year follow-up, and thus in some patients the hyperthermia effect was long-lasting.

This observation was confirmed by Watson et al. (1991) who reported 1 year follow-up on a group of 19 patients treated with the Prostathermer. They found that the increase in flow rate from 7.3 to 10.6 ml/s at 6 week posttherapy was sustained at 1 year and found to be 11.0 ml/s. Symptomatic improvement was also long lasting and remained 50% reduced at 1 year follow-up. This suggests that although no histopathologic change is observed on simple stains, a long-standing change in voiding pattern is obtained in some patients treated with the Prostathermer.

Studies Demonstrating Limited Efficacy

However, not all transrectal hyperthermia trials have demonstrated the same degree of clinical efficacy. Saranga et al. (1990) published a study, also using the Prostathermer, in which 83 severely obstructed patients and 31 patients with indwelling catheters patients were very carefully evaluated and followed. They found that the 83 obstructed patients as a group had symptomatic improvement, but that 37/83 (45%) actually improved and only 18/83 (21%) had greater than a 40% improvement in symptom score. Prostate size was unchanged by hyperthermia treatment alone as determined by transrectal ultrasound, similar to the observation of Lieb et al. (1991b) above. There was no demonstrable statistically significant increase in peak urinary flow rate (10.2 ml/s to 12.1 ml/s at 6 months). Residual urine fell from 130 ml to the statistically significant 56 ml at 12 months posttreatment. When objective and subjective parameters were taken together, they concluded that 28% of patients had successful treatments and 54% were treatment failures. They report an initial 65% (19/29) success in treating urinary retention, but 12 month follow-up included only eight patients. Although many of the patients were selected because they were considered unfit for surgery, the treatments were not without complications. Four patients experienced periprocedure myocardial infarction, and three died. One patient developed intractable hematuria and required immediate prostatectomy. This report suggests that only a small percentage of patients were significantly helped.

Strohmaier et al. (1990) expressed profound disappointment in the technique because it did not combine the advantages of reduced prostatic bulk and increased flow rate seen after successful transurethral prostatic resection (TURP) (Bruskewitz et al. 1986; Meyhoff 1987). Only two of 28 patients (7%) showed improvement comparable to TURP, although 54% of patients did report an overall improved voiding pattern. Follow-up was 4 weeks, and perhaps this did not allow time for the maximal therapeutic effect to be realized. Only one of five patients in retention was freed of his catheters. Similar to the study of Saranga et al. (1990) above, this carefully undertaken study reveals the limits of hyperthermia efficacy.

Other Devices and Applications

In addition to treating a small group with the Prostathermer, Watson et al. (1991) used the Primus prostate machine (Tecnomatix Medical, Belgium) for transrectal hyperthermia treatments on 17 patients. The Primus system uses the same wavelength (915 MHz, treatment at 40 watts) rectal applicator with rectal wall cooling as the Prostathermer, but does not utilize a urethral catheter to measure treatment temperatures. The significance of this difference is that intraprostatic temperatures during treatment are calculated by the device based on the power (wattage) delivered. Investigations by Newman and Knapp (1990) suggest that these temperatures would not be realistic. Certainly, the patient finds the lack of catheterization an advantage, and Watson et al. (1991) treated patients at a target temperature of $42°-44°C$ for six 1 h treatments. They found that the flow rate increases for the Primus-treated group (7.8 ml/s pretreatment to 10.3 ml/s at 6 months) were slightly less than their Prostathermer group (7.3 ml/s pretreatment to 11.0 ml/s at 6 months). Symptomatic improvement was 50% for the Prostathermer group as compared to 40% for the Primus. Again, no change in prostatic volume as determined by ultrasound was reported. Van Erps et al. (1990) reported a preliminary series of 23 patients treated with the Primus prostate machine in which there was a doubling of flow rate 7.9 to 14.3 ml/s after treatment. They found that 56% of patients had objective improvement, and 78% had subjective improvement. Thus, transrectal hyperthermia again is shown to have detectable, even though sometimes variable, beneficial effects on symptomatic BPH.

Although the above review was limited to the treatment of BPH, there are reports to suggest that hyperthermia may have additional clinical applications. Servadio et al. (1987) treated a cohort of 21 patients with symptomatic nonbacterial prostatitis and found many gained relief. In addition, Barnes et al. (1991) observed that many patients with nonbacterial prostatitis or prostatodynia have an erratic flow rate pattern which normalizes after transrectal hyperthermia. This change in voiding dynamics was accompanied by the resolution of painful symptoms attributed to the prostate.

Transrectal Hyperthermia Safety

Transrectal hyperthermia is a relatively safe treatment. In addition to the complications reported above, Lindner et al. (1990b) calculated that of 435 patients treated with the Prostathermer, 27 patients had 29 complications for an overall complication rate of 6.6% Hematuria, infected urine, and epididymitis accounted for 15/29 (51%) of the complications and are likely related to urethral catheterization. This is corroborated by the observation of Watson et al. (1991) that patients treated with the Primus machine who did not undergo catheterization had fewer complications than those treated with the Prostathermer. Chest pain was reported three times, and two patients sustained posttreatment urinary retention. They attribute the fact that none of their patients developed a rectoprostatic fistula to the fact that any patient with an analrectal abnormality was excluded.

Safety of this treatment in sexually active young men was evaluated by Rigatti et al. (1990) who found that neither the morphometric semen analysis nor measurable seminal biochemical constituents were altered by Prostathermer treatment. When compared to the complication rate of TURP, Lindner et al. (1990b) conclude that hyperthermia is an extremely safe treatment.

Summary of Transrectal Hyperthermia

This survey of the transrectal hyperthermia experience allows certain conclusions. The number of transrectal treatments which is necessary for optimum effect is six to ten. The mechanism of action is not known, but the prostate does not seem to undergo a change in volume. There is no rise in posttreatment prostate-specific antigen (PSA) (Lindner et al. 1990c), and this also suggests that there is no cytotoxic effect to the prostatic epithelium. The treatment has a greater impact on the symptoms of outlet obstruction than the objective parameter of peak flow rate. Although all patients are not helped by this treatment, and in some series a strict minority of patients improve, some patients clearly derive some symptomatic benefit from this treatment although their lower urinary tract likely remains obstructed. The subjective or objective improvement obtained by some patients will be maintained up to 1 year or more.

It is currently not possible to explain the variability in response to treatment of the above reported cohorts treated with transrectal hyperthermia. A summary of the responses for patients treated with symptomatic BPH is shown in Table 1, and those treated in retention are summarized in Table 2. Perhaps the small number of treated patients is masking a general pattern. Similarly, patient selection techniques and evaluation may vary between different groups. It is also possible that, although

Table 1. Published series of transrectal hyperthermia treatments for symptomatic BPH

Author (Year)	Instrument (Time/Sessions)	Temperature H (°C)	Patient Number	Parameter	Pretherapy	Posttherapy	Percent Improvement	Follow-up (Months)
Yerushalmi (1985)	Prototype (1 h/7–18)	42–43	18	SYM	9.7	4.1	57%	2–23
Servadio et al. (1987)	Prostathermer (1 h/6–10)	42–43	16	Sym[a] Obj	3.3 14	6.4 27	48% 48%	≤ 24
Servadio et al. (1989)[c]	Prostathermer (1 h/5–10)	39–45	124	PFR PVR SYM[a]	10.1 180 3.8	11.9 90 4.9	18% 50% 29%	6
Saranga et al. (1990)	Prostathermer (1 h/4–7)	42.5	71	PFR PVR SYM[a]	10.2 130 4.6	12.1 56 5.9	28% 19% 57%	6–12
Servadio et al. (1990)[c]	Prostathermer (1/2 - 1 h/6–10)	42	140	OBJ	14–15.5	20–24	47%	12
Strohmaier et al. (1990)	Prostathermer (1 h/8)	42–43	23	PFR PVR SYM	10.9 82 10.7	9.8 75 8.1	−10% 9% 24%	4
Watson et al. (1991)	Prostathermer (1 h/6)	42–44.5	19	PFR PVR SYM	7.3 159 14	10.6 71 7	55% 45% 50%	12
Watson et al. (1991)	Primus (1 h/6)	42–44	17	PFR PVR SYM	7.8 112 13	10.4 30 8	32% 73% 38%	6
Stawarz et al. (1991)	Prototype (1/2 h/6)	42–45	16	PFR SYM	4.5 –[b]	13 –[b]	189% 51%	3

Parameter abreviations: SYM=symptoms score: high=worst, low=best; PFR=peark urinary flow rate in ml/s; PVR=post-void residual urine volume in ml; OBJ=objective score: a mathematical combination of PFR and PVR.

[a] Symptom score: low=worst, high=best.

[b] Symptoms were grouped into levels which do not allow precise determination; 51% of patients improved.

[c] A subset of patients were treated simultaneously with cyproterone acetate.

Table 2. Published series of transrectal hyperthermia treatments for urinary retention

Author (Year)	Instrument (Time/Sessions)	Temperature (°C)	Number of patients in Retention	Patients catheter-free (%)	Follow-up (Months)
Yerushalmi et al. (1985)	Prototype (1 h/4–18)	42–43	11	8 (73)	2–18
Servadio et al. (1987)	Prostathermer (1 h/6–10)	42–43	13	8 (62)	to 24
Lindner et al. (1987)	Prostathermer (1 h/5–10)	39–45	6	5 (85)	to 6
Lindner et al. (1990)[a]	Prostathermer (1 h/3–10)	42	72	36 (50) 29 (40)	1 12
Saranga et al. (1990)	Prostathermer (1 h/8–10)	42.5	29	19 (65)	1
Strohmaier et al. (1990)	Prostathermer (1 h/8)	42	5	1 (20)	1
Stawarz et al. (1991)	Prototype (30 min/6)	42–45	6	4 (67)	3

[a] A subset of patients were simultaneously treated with cyproterone acetate.

similar protocols are followed by different groups, some treatments are more efficacious because the applicator is better aligned with the prostate and thus more heating is obtained. A randomized prospective study is necessary to determine if transrectal hyperthermia is truly efficacious and if so the degree of improvement achieved by patients with BPH.

The Transurethral Thermotherapy Experience

The transrectal approach is relatively inefficient because a significant proportion of the microwave power is lost in the heating the water used to cool the rectal wall. The microwaves have to penetrate tissues with different densities and reflection occurs at interfaces, especially that between the perirectal fat and the prostate. A probe inserted transurethrally can be positioned accurately and easily, leading to confidence that the intended temperature will be achieved in the center of the prostate. A generalized heating profile for a transurethral heating device is shown in Fig. 2a. The temperature is the greatest a short distance from the applicator and falls rapidly as the distance from the urethra is increased. This results in only a small percentage of the prostate receiving maximal therapy. Therefore, some devices have incorporated a circulating cooling fluid to reduce the temperature of the adjacent prostatic urethral wall. The heating profile shown in Fig. 2b demonstrates the addition of cooling by conduction to the heating profile. The device can now emit more power safely and therefore heat a larger volume deeper into the prostate.

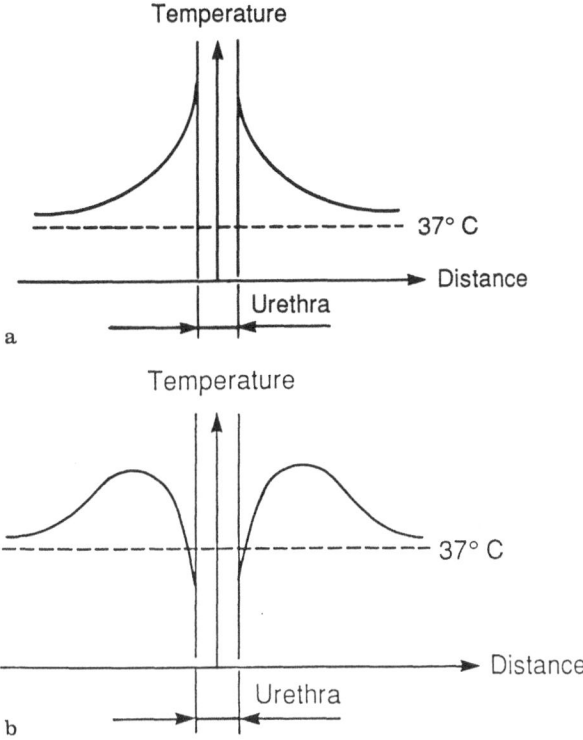

Fig. 2. a The generalized decrease in temperature as distance increases from a transurethral antenna which heats by energy absorption. **b** The summation of cooling by conduction (Fig. 1b) and Fig. 2a showing the combination of transurethral heating by energy absorption and cooling by conduction

Thermotherapy Without Urethral Cooling

Harada et al. (1985, 1987) reported the initial use of a transurethral microwave applicator for prostatic destruction and treated 20 dogs with a 2450 MHz probe at 50 or 100 W for 30 s. Their previous thermal mapping studies demonstrated that when this energy had been delivered to sliced ham, temperatures of 60°C were reached at 50 W and 80°–90°C were reached at 100 W. The treated animals did not require postprocedure catheter drainage, and urethrograms demonstrated an enlarged prostatic urethra. Histopathologic study at 14 days postprocedure showed coagulation and central necrosis of the prostate with fibrous tissue surrounding the injury. Based on the animal studies, the device was determined to be safe and six patients (at least three had prostatic carcinoma) were treated several times at 100 W for 1 min. Five of six patients voided satisfactorily, and posttreatment urethrograms showed an enlarged prostatic fossa. In a larger study, 16 patients with bladder neck obstruction were treated. When compared to 19 patients who underwent a TURP, microwave destruction involved less blood loss and no complications. Sloughing or retention of necrotic prostatic tissue did not occur to a clinically problematic extent. This device requires general anesthesia because of the high temperatures achieved during treatment. In order to treat patients with minimal discomfort at lower temperatures, devices which use lower frequencies have been developed.

A transurethral microwave applicator was described by Astrahan et al. (1989) for intraurethral use at 630 MHz or 915 MHz. Three antennae were symmetrically arranged at 120° intervals around the portion of a modified Foley catheter that is present in the prostatic urethra. Temperature mapping revealed that a well defined area could be heated with excellent ability to control the heating profile. Further mapping studies by Astrahan et al. (1991) revealed that when the urethral feedback thermoregulation is 46°C, a cylindrical volume approximately 4 cm in length and 0.5 cm outward from the device is heated from 47°C to 42°C. The temperature decreases consistently at 6°C/cm. Therefore, no significant temperature increases occur beyond 1 cm and rectal and adjacent organs and neurovascular tissue are not endangered.

Sapozink et al. (1990) used this device (which has been brought to the commercial market by BSD Medical Corp., Salt Lake City, Utah) to treat 21 patients with biopsy proven BPH. The device does not simultaneously cool the adjacent urothelium, and thus creates a cross-sectional heating profile similar to Fig. 2a. Interstitial thermometry revealed that the mean treatment temperature was 44.1°C, the mean maximum temperature was 47.7°C, and maximum temperatures to 49°C were obtained. The histopathologic observations of Lieb et al. (1986) indicate that treatment above 44°C causes areas of prostatic necrosis, and thus treatment above the hyperthermia range has been achieved by this transurethral device and it can be considered to deliver thermotherapy. The mean prostatic volume was 97 ml and patients received ten 1 h treatments over 5 weeks. During or after at least one of the treatment sessions, 71% of patients experienced bladder spasms and hematuria, 48% had dysuria, and 43% experienced urethral pain. The mean duration of follow-up was 12.5 months, and on average the patients had a 44% decrease in nocturia, a 30% increase in the force of stream, a 44% increase in peak flow rate, and a 49% decrease in residual urine volume. Only three patients have needed subsequent prostatectomy to control symptoms.

Using the same transurethral thermotherapy device, the BSD-300 (915 MHz), Baert et al. (1990, 1991) reported treating 15 BPH patients for five to ten 70 min sessions, at 45°C ± 2°. Total symptom score fell from 14.7 to 5.1, prostate volume from 29 to 26 ml, residual urine from 269 to 50 ml, and peak flow rate rose from 6.3 to 12.5 ml/s. All of these changes were statistically significant. The histopathologic examination of tissue of the two patients who needed prostatectomy after a single thermotherapy session revealed early coagulation necrosis extending to 6 mm radially. Chronic bladder atony, prostate asymmetry, and middle lobe configuration were identified as the three patient characteristics that decrease treatment efficacy.

Using a transurethral device similar to the BSD applicator, Stawarz et al. (1991) compared transurethral thermotherapy to transrectal hyperthermia. Transrectal hyperthermia was given at 2450 or 434 MHz using a water-cooled rectal applicator at 42°–45°C for six 30 min treatments. The 2450 MHz transurethral antenna was used for six 30 min treatments at 45°C target temperature. Interstitial thermometry revealed that temperature decreased 3°C per 10 mm distance from the antenna. Although the study was not randomized and transrectal treatments were given to patients treated early in the study, since it was the only available device, the treatment parameters of temperature and time are similar. The reported toxicity was 27% in the transurethral group compared to 8% in the transrectal group. This is similar to the comparative study of Watson et al. (1991). There was significant increase in flow rate and decrease in postvoid residual in both groups, but in these categories neither method was statistically superior to the other. However, the transurethral-treated group had a 79% improvement in symptomatology, statistically superior to the 41% improvement in the transrectal group. Prostate volume, although not determined exactly, seemed to decrease by more than reported in any other study in both groups. Patients with large median prostatic lobes, which are often intravesicular, accounted for 61% of transrectal failures and 100% of transurethral failures. This is understandable since the transurethral antenna is not in contact with the larger middle lobe, and similar findings have been reported by other groups.

Thermotherapy with Urethral Cooling

In order to obtain higher treatment temperatures throughout more of the prostate, transurethral cooling can be added to the transurethral antenna unit. Since pain becomes more pronounced when the prostatic urothelium is heated to over 46°C, the Prostatron (Technomed International) was developed to destroy tissue deeper within the prostate by heat treatment of 45°–55°C while preserving the urothelium. Deconec et al. (1991) demonstrated that in order to obtain tissue destruction from heating 10–15 mm deep into the prostate from a urethral microwave antenna, the urethral wall would need to be heated to 75°–80°C. This underscores the need for periurethral cooling if local anesthesia is used. The heating distribution of the Prostatron approximates that shown in Fig. 2b, and tissue destruction occurs in any zone heated to >45°C for more than 30 min. Devonec et al. (1991) undertook clinical trials in which the 1296 MHz applicator was used to heat prostates to measured temperatures of 45°–55°, while computer-controlled feedback loops maintain energy output so the urethra was <44.5°C and the rectal wall was <42.5°C. Histopathology of treated glands revealed that the urethral mucosa was preserved to a depth of 2–5 mm, and that necrosis was obtained at a distance from 5 to 17 mm from the luminal antenna. A total of 37 patients were treated with transurethral lidocaine for anesthesia with a single 55 min session. This treatment time is based on their findings that temperatures >45°C are obtained with 15–20 min of initiating treatment and that at least 30 min at thermotherapy temperature is necessary for tissue destruction. The treatment occurs in three phases during the 55 min. First the urethra is cooled, and the microwave emission begins at a maximum of 55 W or until the rectal temperature reaches 42.5°C. The urethral temperature is then allowed to rise to a maximum of 44.5°C. The 3 month follow-up on this cohort of patients revealed that the symptom score fell from 12 to 8 ($p = 0.006$), peak flow rate increased from 8.4 to 10.8 ml/s ($p = 0.030$), residual urine fell from 109 to 50 ml ($p = 0.043$). Prostatic volume did not change (mean 53 ml). PSA was found to increase from 4.2 to 11.3 1 week after treatment. Once again, there is a larger impact on symptoms than flow rate, and the increase in PSA is consistent with tissue destruction.

In an adjunctive study, Carter et al. (1991) treated 50 patients with the Prostatron, but in one patient the catheter could not be successfully passed and in a second the applicator failed. In a group of 19 Prostatron-treated patients in retention with an indwelling catheter, six (32%) were voiding (follow-up 6 weeks to 5 months), seven have undergone TURP, two remain with a catheter, and one died. Another group of 23 patients with normal detrusor function and prostatic outlet obstruction was treated with the Prostatron. Peak flow rate increased from 8.2 to 14.3 ml/s at 3 month follow-up, and most patients had symptomatic improvement. The average pretreatment prostatic urethral length, which was measured by ultrasound to be 44 mm, decreased more than 6 mm in 31% of patients at 6 weeks and in 57% of patients at 12 weeks. This observation indicates that structural remodeling of the prostate continues to occur for at least 12 weeks. Patients with the greatest increase in flow rate also had maximal shortening of the prostatic urethra. As is often the case after thermotherapy, the authors note that there was a transient worsening of irritative and obstructive symptoms during the first few days after treatment. This finding is attributed to edema of the prostatic adenoma brought about by the inflammatory response.

Perez-Castro et al. (1991) reported on 100 patients treated with the Prostatron. The patient cohort responded similar to that of Carter et al. (1991), and the authors attempted to more carefully define the selection criteria for hyperthermia treatment. They concluded that the beneficial treatment response is highest in a patient less than 70 years old with a prostatic urethra less than 45–50 mm in echographic length, a median prostatic lobe which is not hypertrophied, and good bladder contractility as demonstrated by no history of urinary retention or a large postvoid residual urine volume.

Other Thermotherapy Devices

The Thermex-II (Direx LTD, Israel) is a transurethral prostatic heating device which utilizes capacitative diathermy, not a microwave antenna, to heat the prostate. An electrode mounted on a modified urethral catheter is placed in the prostate and a metal plate is fixed to each inner upper thigh. This device heats the prostatic urothelium adjacent to the heating element to 44.5°C for a single 3 h session. Histologic examination of canine prostate 1 week after Thermex-II treatment reveals that the urethral epithelium is regenerated and that there is capillary bleeding and mononuclear cell infiltration (Meshorer 1990). At 1 month posttreatment, there are decreased glandular elements. Watson et al. (1991) treated 12 BPH patients with the device and found peak flow rate was statistically unchanged at 6 weeks posttherapy having increased from 11.2 ml/s to 12.8 ml/s. However, they note that the symptom score decreased from 13 to 8 (38%). In a patient who came to TURP, histopathology revealed infarction of the periurethral prostate. This suggests this device has a larger impact on symptoms than objective parameters, similar to the observation of Stawarx et al. (1991).

In a larger series, van den Bossche et al. (1991) treated 62 patients with the Thermex-II. At 2 month follow-up, 77% (17/22) had subjective improvement and 32% (7/22) had greater than a 50% increase in flow rate. They observed that the PSA was two- to three-fold higher on the day following therapy, and returned to pretherapy levels at 1 month. There was no change in volume as measured by ultrasound, an observation also reported by Watson et al. (1991), and no change was seen on magnetic resonance imaging. Their histopathologic examination revealed the maximum periurethral necrotic area to be $15 \times 10 \times 10$ mm. Epithelial regeneration of the prostatic fossa had occurred.

In order to obtain greater tissue destruction, higher temperatures can be used. Prostatic heat treatments to $80°-90°C$ have been undertaken in the canine prostate using a 7 French catheter which was heat emitting, computer-controlled, and could be placed in the prostatic urethra. This method of Castaneda et al. (1991) heats completely by conduction and could reliably debulk the central periurethral adenoma in a controlled manner. Retrograde urethrography 1 month after treatment demonstrated a enlarged prostatic urethra, and this is confirmed on gross and microscopic pathologic examination. The authors suggest that this treatment may be offered in the outpatient setting since there is no bleeding, and urinary retention may not occur if the sloughing occurs slowly.

Summary of Transurethral Thermotherapy

Transurethral devices do have the potential of causing necrosis and, therefore, of acting on both the static and the dynamic component of the prostatic obstruction. The transurethral systems are slightly more invasive than the transrectal devices that only use a rectal applicator (Primus Prostate Machine); however most transrectal devices have transurethral temperature monitors and most transurethral devices have transrectal temperature sensors. The addition of the transurethral cooling component by the Prostatron allowed higher intraprostatic temperatures to be reached during a local anesthetic procedure. However, it has not been demonstrated that preserving the prostatic urothelium decreased the incidence of post-procedure sloughing, leading to urinary retention or bleeding, and was in fact essential for a successful outcome.

The transurethral thermotherapy experience in treating symptomatic BPH is summarized in Table 3, and those patients presenting with urinary retention are summarized in Table 4. Transurethral thermotherapy has been demonstrated to be more effective in producing symptomatic relief than increasing peak urinary flow rate. Patients who have decreased detrusor function or a large middle prostatic lobe have a decreased chance of obtaining a response. Since the prostatic urethra continues to undergo remodeling for up to 3 months after thermotherapy, it is not possible to assess maximal beneficial effect until that time. The transurethral technology is too new to assess the long-term effects and whether the improvement obtained by some patients will be long-lasting.

Table 3. Published series of transurethral thermotherapy treatments for symptomatic BPH

Author (Year)	Instrument (Time/Sessions)	Temperature (°C)	Patient Number	Parameter	Pre-therapy	Post-therapy	Percent Improvement
Sapozink et al. (1990)	Prototype (1 h/up to 10)	44 (41–47)	21	FRE	2.4	2.8	−16%
				NOC	3.7	2.1	43%
				PFR	11.0	15.9	45%
				PVR	177	91	49%
Baert et al. (1990)	BSD (70 min/5–10)	45	12	PFR	6.3	12.5	99%
				PVR	269	50	80%
				SYM	14.7	5.1	65%
Stawarz et al. (1991)	BSD (30 min/3–6)	47	10	PFR	3.8	9.0	136%
				SYM	−[a]	−[a]	79%
Van den Bossche et al. (1991)	Thermex-II (3 h/1)	44.5	22	PFR	−[b]	−[b]	32%–43%
				PVR	−[c]	−[c]	27%–43%
				SYM	−[d]	−[d]	57%–77%
Watson et al. (1991)	Thermex-II (3 h/1)	44.5	12	PFR	11.2	12.8	14%
				PVR	71	29	59%
				SYM	13	8	38%
Devonec et al. (1991)	Prostatron (55 min/1)	>45.5	37	PFR	8.4	10.8	29%
				PVR	109	50	54%
				SYM	12	8	33%
Carter et al. (1991)	Prostatron (55 min/1)	>44.5	23	PFR	8.2	14.3	74%
				PVR	64	58	13%
				SYM	−[e]	−[e]	100%

SYM symptom score high=worst, low=best; FRE daytime frequency; NOC, nocturia; PFR, peak flow rate in ml/s; PVR postvoid residual in ml; OBJ, mathematical combination of PFR and PVR.
[a]Symptoms were grouped into levels which do not allow for precise determination. 79% of patients improved.
[b]PFR data reveals that from 32%–43% of patients had >50% increase in flow rate.
[c]PVR data reveals that from 27%–43% of patients had >50% decrease in residual urine volume.
[d]Symptoms were not reported exactly other than 57%–77% of patients improved.
[e]Symptoms were not reported exactly other than all patients had improvement at 6 and 12 week follow-up.

Table 4. Published series of transurethral thermotherapy treatments for urinary retention

Author (Year)	Instrument (Time/Sessions)	Temp (°C)	Patients in Retention	Patients catheter-free (%)	Follow-up (Months)
Baert et al. (1990)	BSD (70 min/5–10)	45	3	1 (33)	1–3
Stawarz et al. (1991)	BSD (30 min/3–6)	47	4	1 (25)	3
Van den Bossche et al. (1991)	Thermex-II (3 h/1)	44.5	17	8 (47)	1 week
Carter et al. (1991)	Prostatron (55 min/1)	>45.5	19	6 (32)	1 1/2–5

The Role of Prostatic Heat Treatments in Therapy

Benign prostatic hypertrophy originates in the transition and periurethral zones of the prostate. However, only approximately 50% of patients with microscopic BPH will develop macroscopic BPH, and only 50% of patients with macroscopic BPH will have symptoms necessitating intervention (see recent review by Osterling 1991). Prostatic obstruction has two components: the static component of urethral blockage by the adenoma and the dynamic component of prostatic smooth muscle. Until recently, intervention was synomous with prostatectomy, and the probability that a 50 year old man would undergo a prostatectomy in his lifetime was estimated to be 25%–35%. The development of new less invasive therapies will likely bring many additional patients to treatment since the risks associated with the new therapies are less than those of prostatectomy.

Approximately 80% of prostatectomies are performed in the United States for symptoms; and it is the symptoms that usually first bring a patient to the urologist. The irritative and obstructive symptoms of prostatism are related to the obstruction-induced changes in bladder function. The irritative symptoms of frequency and urgency, often the most bothersome to patients, result from detrusor instability. The second obstruction-induced change in bladder function is decreased detrusor contractility, and this results in the obstructive symptoms of decreased force of stream, intermittency, and increased residual urine.

There are a number of issues raised when considering any new modality for the treatment of BPH. The evaluation of the heat treatment trials and the comparison of different devices needs to include assessment of the validity of the outcome indicators, the placebo effect, and the natural history of the disease being studied. In order to compare the many new devices, similar outcome indicators must be available for analysis. Unfortunately, often the many different groups undertaking investigations into device efficacy report the data in a manner which makes direct comparison difficult. In general, there are two groups of outcome indicators: objective parameters and subjective symptoms. The objective parameters are features of voiding that can be numerically measured, i.e., peak urinary flow rate and postvoid residual urine volume. The symptoms a patient experiences are considered subjective, even though a numerical assessment of their severity can be compiled.

Evaluation of Outcome Indicators

One of the most commonly reported objective parameters is increase in peak urinary flow rate. This parameter, to be maximally valid as an outcome indicator, should be reported for an average of several representative voids and reported with the total voided volume and postvoid residual (Siroky et al. 1979; Siroky 1990). Flowmetry is not reliable for a total voided volume less than 150 ml, and flow rate varies for an individual when different volumes are voided. Since this type of detailed flow rate analysis is not reported in the prostatic heat treatment reports, comparison between studies is very difficult, and even the interpretation of the absolute increase in flow rate reported in any individual study must take this shortcoming into account. Further complicating the interpretation of reported flowmetry is that some studies do not report exact increases in flow rate, but rather report that a certain percentage of patients had a specified increase which the author has chosen as significant. Only a general conclusion can be reached, and that is some patients experience an increase in flow rate after treatment and that increase is often 2–4 ml/s. The impact that this increase in flow has on the patients quality of life and its clinical and pathophysiologic significance is unclear.

The other commonly measured objective parameter is postvoid residual volume, and there is an improvement in this parameter in almost all hyperthermia and thermotherapy trials in which it is determined. Although a decrease in this volume should be associated with better bladder emptying, there is as yet no evidence of changed urodynamic bladder measurements after treatment which would support this concept. It is possible that the better bladder emptying which many patients achieve will reduce the chance of urinary infection and protect against detrusor failure and upper tract deterioration.

The patient usually seeks therapeutic intervention because of his symptoms, and therefore symptom assessment is extremely important. A number of different symptom scoring systems exist to quantitate the voiding experience of the patient. Many of the studies created their own scoring systems, and others used the published systems of Boyarksy et al. (1977) or Madsen and Iverson (1983). The patient response to a symptom score depends on whether it is self-administered or administered by a health professional. The use of disparate scoring systems by the different studies does not allow direct comparison between the hyperthermia and thermotherapy techniques, nor among the devices with a single group. However, the overall pattern evident from all of the studies taken together is that there is a major impact on symptoms, often in excess of the improvement seen in the objective parameters.

Role of the Placebo Effect

The second issue raised when evaluating this new modality is the placebo effect encountered in BPH treatment. The placebo effect is well known, and Resnick et al. (1983) demonstrated a statistically significant improvement in subjective symptoms and peak urinary flow rate in a placebo group participating in a controlled drug study for the treatment of BPH. In addition, flow rate increases were noted during the lead-in study time before drug was given in the finasteride study (MK-906 Study Group 1991). Issacs (1990) analyzed the placebo effect in controlled drug trials and concluded that it is usually not prolonged and symptoms tend to revert to baseline by 6 months. This argues that there is a placebo effect in the patients treated with the heating devices, but that follow-up for greater than 6 months should diminish its importance. Therefore, the placebo contribution to reported treatment effects in studies of short follow-up cannot be assessed, and it may be a major component of the response. However, the flow rate increases of 4–5 ml/s reported in some patient subgroups after thermotherapy treatment are in excess of those expected from placebo if no physical intervention had taken place, and therefore are at least partially due to the intervention. Since no study to date has inserted the urethral or rectal probes without activating the heating elements, it cannot be unequivocally stated that the effect seen in flow rate is in excess of a true placebo control for the device.

Role of the Natural History of BPH

The third and final aspect of the evaluation of heat therapy is consideration of the natural history of the disease and the impact of treatment on that natural history. Issacs (1990) has reviewed the small number of existing papers on the natural history of BPH and found that approximately 20% of patients tend to improve and 20% tend to deteriorate after initial evaluation. The course of the disease waxes and wanes for the remaining 60%. Issacs concluded that those patients who have the greatest degree of spontaneous improvement usually have had a history of symptoms of less than 6 months. It is hard to evaluate the impact of heat treatment on this natural history, although it seems clear that more than 20% of some of the study groups improve, and this is in excess of what might be expected without intervention. Most of the studies have at least 20% of patients who fail to improve, and it is possible that the heat treatments are not successful in changing the natural history for that group which is destined to deteriorate. However, for the 60% of patients who are likely not to experience a spontaneous improvement, the heat treatments in many of the trials seem adequately efficacious to improve the quality of life for many of these individuals.

The eventual role of prostatic heat treatments in the urologists rapidly expanding number of treatment options for BPH is not yet determined. As devices become more sophisticated, it may be possible to obtain more tissue destruction in an outpatient ambulatory setting. This new technology may offer long-standing relief to carefully selected patients.

References

Astrahan MA, Sapozink MD, Cohen D, Luxton G, Kampp TD, Boyd S, Petrovich Z (1989) Microwave applicator for transurethral hyperthermia of benign prostatic hyperplasia. Int J Hyperthermia 5:283–296

Astrahan MA, Ameye F, Oyen R, Willeman P, Baert L, Petrovich Z (1991) Interstitial temperature measurements during transurethral microwave hyperthermia. J Urol 145:304–308

Baert L, Ameye F, Willemen P, Vandenhove J, Lauweryns J, Astrahan M, Petrovich Z (1990) Transurethral microwave hyperthermia for benign prostatic hyperplasia: preliminary clinical and pathological results. J Urol 144:1383–1387

Baert L, Willeman P, Ameye F, Petrovich Z (1991) Treatment response with transurethral microwave hyperthermia in different froms of bening prostatic hyperplasia: a preliminary report. Prostate 18:315–320

Barnes DG, Perlmutter AP, Watson GM (1991) Transrectal hyperthermia in the benign painful prostate. World J Urol 9:12–14

Bosch RJLH, Griffiths DJ, Blom JHM, Schroeder FH. (1989) Treatment of benign prostatic hyperplasia by androgen deprivation: effects on prostate size and urodynamic parameters. J Urol 141:68

Boyarsky S, Jones G, Paulson DF, Prout GR (1977) A new look at bladder neck obstruction by the Food and Drug Administration regulators: guidelines for investigation of benign prostatic hypertrophy. Trans Am Assoc Genito Urinary Surg 68:29-32

Bruskewitz RC, Larsen EH, Madsen PO, Dorflinger T (1986) Three year follow-up of urinary symptoms after transurethral resection of the prostate. J Urol 136:613

Busch W (1866) Über den Einfluss, welchen heftigere Erysipeln zuweilen auf organisierte Neubildungen ausüben. Verhandl Naturh Preus, Rhein Westphal 23:28

Caine M, Perlberg S, Meretyk S (1978) A placebo-controlled double-blind study of the effect of phenoxybenzamine in benign prostatic obstruction. Br J Urol 50:551

Carter SSC, Patel A, Reddy P, Royer P, Ramsay JWA (1991) Single-session transurethral microwave thermotherapy for the treatment of benign prostatic obstruction. J Endourol 5:137-144

Castaneda F, Banno J, Brady T (1991) Experimental prostatic hyperthermia. J Endourol 5:123-127

Devonec M, Berger N, Perrin P (1991) Transurethral microwave heating of the prostate- or from hyperthermia to thermotherapy. J Endourol 5:129-135

Harada T, Etori K, Kumazaki T, Nishizawa O, Noto H, Tsuchda S (1985) Microwave surgical treatment of diseases of the prostate. Urology 26:572-576

Harada T, Tsuchida S, Nishizana O et al. (1987) Microwave surgical treatment of the prostate: clinical application of microwave surgery as a tool for improved prostatic electroresection. Urol Int 42:127-131

Issacs JT (1990) Importance of the natural history of benign prostatic hyperplasia in the evaluation of pharmacologic intervention. Prostate Suppl 3:1-7

Katzir A, Bowman HF, Asfour Y, Zur A, Valeri CR (1989) Infared fibers for radiometer themometry in hypothermia and hyperthermia treatment. Trans Biomed Eng 36:634-637

Lieb Z, Rothem A, Lev A, Servadio C (1986) Histopatholocal observations in the canine prostate treated by local microwave hyperthermia. Prostate 8:93-102

Lieb, Z, Lev A, Goren E, Servadio C (1991a) Observations on the influence of syproterone acetate on the sonographic image of the begin prostate in patients treated with local hyperthermia. World J Urol 9:19-21

Lieb Z, Lev A, Servadio C (1991b) Transrectal ultrasound in local hyperthermia to the benign prostate. World J Urol 9:15-18

Lindner A, Golomb J, Siegel Y, Lev A (1987) Local hyperthermia of the prostate gland for the treatment of benign prostatic hypertrophy and urinary retention: a preliminary report. Br J Urol 60:567-571

Lindner A, Braf Z, Lev A, Golumb J, Leib Y, Siegel Y, Servadio C (1990a) Local hyperthermia of the prostate gland for the treatment of benign prostatic hypertrophy and urinary retention. Br J Urol 65:201-203

Lindner A, Siegel R, Saranga R, Korzcak D, Matzkin H, Braf Z (1990b) Complications in hyperthermia treatment of benign prostatic hyperplasia. J Urol 144:1390-1392

Lindner A, Siegel YI, Korczak D (1990c) Serum prostatic specific antigen levels during hyperthermia treatment of benign prostatic hyperplasia. J Urol 144:1388-1389

Madsen OM Iverson P (1983) A point system for selecting operative candidates. In: Hinman F Jr (ed) Benign Prostatic Hypertrophy. Springer, Berlin Heidelberg New York, p 763

Magin RL, Fridd CW, Bonfiglio TA Linke CA (1980) Thermal destruction of the canine prostate by high intensity microwaves. J Surg Res 29:265-275

Matsuda H, Sugimachi K, Kuwano H, Mori M (1989) Hyperthermia, tissue microcirculation, and temporarily increased thermosensitivity in VX2 carcinoma in rabbit liver. Cancer Res 49:2777-2782

Meshorer A (1990) Treatment of BPH using the Thermex-II. Abstracts Eur Assoc Urol IX Congr 18 [Suppl 1]:264

Meyhoff H-H (1987) Transurethral versus transvesical prostatectomy. clinical, urodynamic, renographic, and economic aspects a randomized study. Scand J Nephrol [Suppl] 102:1-26

MK-906 (Finasteride) Study Group (1991) One-year experience in the treatment of benign prostatic hyperplasia with finasteride. J Androl 12:372-375

Newman D, Knapp P (1990) Interstitial temperature mapping in human prostate during transrectal hyperthermia treatment for BPH. J Endourol 4:S135

Nishimura Y, Jo S, Akuta K, Masunaga S, Fushiki M, Hiraoka M, Takahashi M, Abe M (1989) Histological analysis of the effect of hyperthermia on normal rat hepatic vasculature. Cancer Res 49:4295-4297

Osterling JE (1991) The origin and development of benign prostatic hyperplasia: and age dependent process. J Androl 12:348-355

Paliwal BR, Shrivastava PN (1989) Microwave hyperthermia: principles and quality assurance. Radiol Clin North Am 27:489-497

Perez-Castro E, Carbonero M, Mancebo JM, Massarra J, Iglesias JI (1991) Tratamiento de la hipertrofia benigna prostatica (HPB) con termoterapia transurettal. Experiencia inicial. Arch Esp Urol 44.5:637-645

Resnick MI, Jackson JE, Watts LE, Boyce WH (1983) Assessment of the antihypercholesterolemic drug, probucol, in benign prostatic hyperplasia. J Urol 129:206-209

Rigatti P, Buonaguidi A, Grasso M, Lania C, Montorsi F, Colombo R, Galli L, Guazzoni G. (1990) Morphometric and biochemical assessment of seminal plasma in patients who underwent local prostatic hyperthermia. Prostate 16:325-330

Sapareto SA, Dewy WC (1984) Thermal dose determination in cancer therapy. J Radiat Oncol Biol Phys 10:787-800

Sapozink MD, Boyd SD, Astrahan MA, Jozsef G, Petrovich Z. (1990) Transurethral hyperthermia for benign prostatic hyperplasia: preliminary clinical results. J Urol 113:944-950

Saranga R, Matzkin H, Braf Z (1990) Local microwave hyperthermia in the treatment of benign prostatic hyperplasia. Br J Urol 65:349-353

Servadio C, Leib Z, (1984) Hyperthermia in the treatment of prostate cancer. Prostate 5:205-211

Servadio C, Lieb Z, Lev A (1986) Further observations on the use of local hyperthermia for the treatment of diseases of the prostate in man. Eur J Urol 12:38-40

Servadio C, Leib Z, Lev A (1987) Diseases of prostate treated by local microwave hyperthermia. Urology 30:97-99

Servadio C, Linder A, Lev A, Leib Z, Siegel Y, Braf Z (1989) Further observations on the effect of local hyperthermia on benign enlargement of the prostate. World J Urol 6:204-208

Servadio C, Braf Z, Siegel Y, Leib Z, Saranga R, Lindner A. (1990) Local thermotherapy of the benign prostate: a 1-year follow-up. Eur Urol 18:169-173

Siroky MB (1990) Interpretation of urinary flow rates. Urol Clin North Am 17:537-542

Siroky MB, Olsson C, Krane RJ (1979) The flow rate nomogram: I. Development. J Urol 122:665-668

Song CW (1978) Effect of hyperthermia on vascular functions of normal tissues and experimental tumours. JNCI 60:711-713

Stawarz B, Szmiglielski S, Orgrodnik J, Astrahan M, Petrovich Z (1991) A comparison of transurethral and transrectal microwave hyperthermia in poor risk surgical benign prostatic hypertrophy patients. J Urol 146:353-357

Strohmaier WL, Bichler KH, Fluchter SH, Wilbert DM (1990) Local microwave hyperthermia of benign prostatic hyperplasia. J Urol 144:913-917

Van den Bossche M, Noel JC, Schulman CC (1991) Transurethral hyperthermia for benign prostatic hypertrophy. World J Urol 9:2-6

Van Erps P, Dourcy B, Denis LJ (1990) Transrectal hyperthermia in benign prostatic hyperplasia (BPH. Abstr Eur Assoc Urol IX Congr 18 [Suppl 1]:510

Watson GM, Perlmutter AP, Shah TK, Barnes DG (1991) Heat treatment for severe, symptomatic prostatic outflow obstruction. World J Urol 9:7-11

Yerushalmi A (1975) Cure of a solid tumor by simultaneous administration of microwaves and x-ray irradiation. Radiat Res 64:602

Yerushalmi A, Servadio C, Leib Z, Fishelovitz Y, Rokowsky E, Stein JA (1982) Local hyperthermia for treatment of carcinoma of the prostate: a preliminary report. Prostate 3:623-630

Yerushalmi A, Fishelovitz Y, Singer D, Reiner I, Arielly J, Abramovici Y, Catsenelson R, Levy E, Shani A (1985) Localized deep microwave hyperthermia in the treatment of poor operative risk patients with benign prostatic hyperplasia. J Urol 133:873-876

Laser Prostatectomy*

R.A.Roth

Introduction

Lasers have several useful properties for the treatment of patients with prostatic obstruction. Laser energy can be delivered through small endoscopes and laser energy can destroy prostate tissue while producing hemostasis. Because perioperative bleeding is the major cause of morbidity associated with prostatectomy, a technique that minimizes or eliminates bleeding could reduce morbidity, hospitalization, and costs and, therefore, improve outcome of prostatectomy. For a laser to be truly useful in treating prostatic obstruction, it also must be capable of removing substantial amounts of tissue to relieve anatomic obstruction.

Previous attempts (Cohen and Warner 1988; Shanberg et al. 1985; Silber and Servadio 1991) at neodymium:yttrium aluminum garnet (Nd:YAG) laser prostatectomy have met with varied results. Most of these techniques used a laser cystoscope to deliver energy. This instrument is a standard cystoscope with a slightly modified Albarran bridge to deflect the laser fiber at 30°–40° angle to the long axis. This device was originally designed for the treatment of bladder tumors and is not optimal for treating narrow tubular structures, such as the prostate (Hofstetter 1986). A urologist performs prostatectomy with this device by inserting the fiber directly into the obstructing tissue and firing the laser long enough to cause tissue vaporization. Since the laser fibers are usually 0.4–0.6 mm in diameter and the area of tissue loss is only somewhat larger, it is time-consuming to remove a substantial amount of tissue. With persistence, prostate tissue can be ablated, and hemostasis is usually adequate. Clinical reports indicate that obstruction is relieved and patients tolerate the procedure well. Because of the time and effort involved, however, this method holds small advantage over standard electrosurgical means.

The Nd:YAG laser has been used more commonly in conjunction with extensive transurethral resection of the prostate to treat carcinoma of the prostate gland. After a suitable postoperative recovery period, the residual prostatic tissue is irradiated with the laser to destroy all residual prostatic tissue. Because of the way the laser cystoscope is designed, it is difficult to see and radiate the acute angles of the apical

*This work is supported by IntraSonix, Inc., Burlington, Massachusetts, in which the Lahey Clinic and the author have a minority financial interest.

areas, and it is necessary to use an endoscope passed antegrade through a suprapubic cannula for complete treatment. Preliminary results indicate that excellent control of tumor can be achieved with this method (Beisland and Sander 1986; McNicholas 1988).

Recently, a side-firing laser fiber has been developed to improve on the ability to deliver the laser into a tubular structure (Costello and Johnson 1991; Johnson et al. 1991 a,b). This fiber can be placed through a conventional endoscope under direct vision and can be used to treat and remove obstructing tissue. Results of early clinical studies are currently not available, but theoretically this technique may have an advantage of simplicity in that conventional instrumentation and direct vision can be used.

An ideal laser device should cause instant efficient ablation of tissue and complete coagulation of blood vessels. Present laser technology and instrumentation do not meet this ideal, but a laser delivery system has been developed that overcomes many of the deficiencies of the standard laser cystoscope. A practical laser delivery system should have low capital outlay and disposable equipment costs, be durable, be minimally invasive and able to be introduced into the prostate gland with ease, permit treatment based on individual prostate anatomy, have a reliable outcome, have precise depth of laser delivery control, and have a short learning curve. With these needs in mind, a new laser delivery system for relief of prostatic obstruction was devised.

The Transurethral Ultrasound-Guided Laser-Induced Prostatectomy System

In 1988, urologists at the Lahey Clinic Medical Center and engineers at IntraSonix, Inc., Burlington, Massachusetts, were the first to conceive and develop a new laser delivery system that includes a side-firing Nd:YAG laser that is guided by real-time ultrasonography instead of endoscopic vision (Roth et al. 1990). Both the ultrasound waves and laser energy pass through a balloon positioned in the lumen of the prostate gland. The balloon is invisible to the laser beam and the ultrasound waves and remains in place and intact throughout the procedure.

It is useful to review some of the effects of Nd:YAG laser energy on tissue and how this energy is delivered to understand the construction and use of the transurethral ultrasound-guided laser-induced prostatectomy (TULIP)[TM]* system (IntraSonix, Inc.). At a wavelength of 1064 nm, Nd:YAG laser energy can be transmitted through semiflexible quartz fibers through both rigid and flexible endoscopes. Laser light at 1064 nm is poorly absorbed by water, meaning that the light will pass through water or waterlike tissues with little absorption. Because of this property,

---

* TULIP is a trademark of IntraSonix, Inc.

the light can penetrate relatively deeply into tissue and, when converted to thermal energy, will create substantial tissue damage. Dosimetry studies (Newman and Jacques 1991) have shown that the Nd:YAG laser will penetrate into tissue 4–6 mm, whereas the carbon dioxide (CO_2) laser with high water absorption characteristics will penetrate only a fraction of 1 mm. The mechanism of tissue injury is the conversion of light to thermal energy or heat. In terms of quantification, the amount of laser energy introduced is in watts (W), the duration of the light is in terms of seconds, and the product becomes measurement of delivered heat or joules (J).

In living tissue, a dynamic relationship occurs between the amount of energy that is absorbed by the tissue, the amount of heat dissipated by conduction, and the amount of heat that is carried off by the blood vessels. The result is a net rise in tissue temperature. When the temperature is raised to 40°–50°C, little permanent damage occurs in the tissue. At 50°–100°C, proteins are denatured, although the tissue structurally remains intact and coagulation necrosis occurs. When 100°C is exceeded, tissue fluid boils and results in small explosions causing disruption and vaporization, which is known as the "popcorn" effect (Fisher 1987).

In endoscopic procedures, laser energy can be delivered either by direct contact or by a noncontact mode. In the former, the tip of the fiber is pushed into the tissue, and the laser actuated. A rapid rise in tissue temperature to 100°C occurs, and popcorn explosions result with vaporization and mechanical destruction of tissue. Because laser fibers are typically 0.4–0.6 mm in diameter and the popcorn effect is not much more than 1 mm, a good deal of time is needed to effect any substantial amount of tissue destruction. Charring of the fiber tip is common, thus limiting laser tissue penetration, and hemostasis is not complete because blood vessels and tissue are disrupted. For these reasons, a direct contact means of destroying the prostate gland shows no great advantage over conventional electrosurgical devices.

In the noncontact mode, the laser fiber is held away from the tissue, and the tissue is irradiated from a constant distance (Frank 1988). This has the advantage of keeping a clean noncharred tip and minimizes popcorn explosions. The farther the fiber tip is held away from the tissue, the less focused the beam and the less penetration. Thus, variation in standoff causes a variable delivered dose. Another factor that decreases absorption is the presence of blood on the tissue surface. Blood readily absorbs Nd:YAG laser energy and prevents deep penetration.

When tissue is coagulated by the noncontact mode, it tends to shrink and turn white. It is well known in laser surgery that thermal effects apparent on the tissue surface do not necessarily reflect the net heat damage within the tissue. In prostate tissue treated with the Nd:YAG laser, an inverted mushroom-shaped tissue injury typically occurs, with the cap facing the capsule of the prostate gland and the stem toward the lumen of the prostate gland. It is not possible to tell by endoscopic visualization alone during laser irradiation how deeply or extensively laser energy is penetrating beneath the surface of the tissue nor is it possible to estimate the thickness of the tissue to be irradiated. Although control of laser dose is an important factor in the effective and safe delivery of laser energy, control is difficult to achieve with endoscopic or direct visualization alone.

The TULIP system was designed to deliver Nd:YAG laser energy uniformly, efficiently, and safely into the prostate gland. The device is composed of a 20 French metal probe with a 600 μm fused silica laser fiber at one end that is coupled to a microprism (Fig. 1). This prism is able to bend the laser light at a 90° angle to the long axis of the probe, thus enabling irradiation of any part of the lumen of the prostate gland from apex to bladder neck. On either side of the laser prism is a miniaturized ultrasound transducer that creates a 90° sector scan at 7.5 MHz. The transducer is constructed so that the laser beam always transects the exact middle of the ultrasound scan so that targeted tissue is always in the center of the ultrasound picture. The ultrasound scan can be adjusted from 2 mm to 5 cm in depth, permitting any prostate gland to be seen from its lumen to the capsule and beyond.

The real-time ultrasound scan guides the laser treatment (Fig. 2). Instead of using direct vision to determine anatomic landmarks for where to start and where to stop laser treatment, the ultrasound picture identifies these landmarks but also has the added dimension of being able to see the depth of the prostate gland at any point along the urethra. Without this extra dimension, how much energy should be directed into any specific area cannot be estimated. When tissue depth is not known, laser irradiation is performed based on guess and results of animal dosimetry studies, and thus overtreatment or undertreatment is just as likely to result as optimal treatment. Using the TULIP ultrasound, the urologist can look at the scan and determine where to start and stop laser delivery as well as to adjust the speed (seconds) of the laser traverse, thereby controlling absorbed energy and tissue

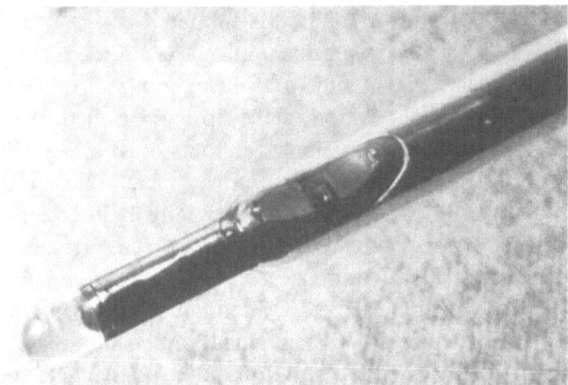

Fig. 1. TULIP probe; tip of 20 French metal probe. Laser microprism bends laser at 90° to long axis of probe a split ultrasound transducer is on either side of prism. The ultrasound transducer oscillates back and forth to create a 90° sector scan. Laser prism is fixed in position in exact center of ultrasound transducer and scan. (From Roth and Aretz 1991)

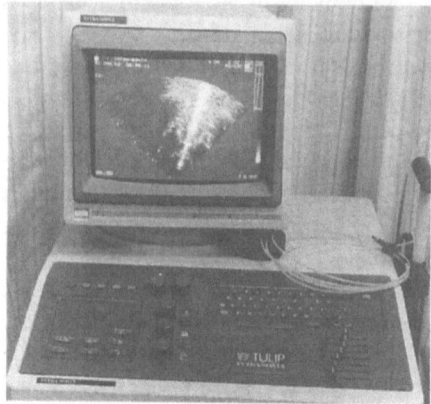

Fig. 2. TULIP ultrasound control and screen

damage. In addition, the ultrasound transducer can determine textural differences and anatomic zones, the presence of calculi and blood vessels, and perhaps the amount of adenomatous versus stromal tissue within the prostate gland. These factors may permit even greater individualization of treatment to be devised.

To deliver the laser energy effectively and to obtain a satisfactory ultrasound image, the transducer and laser prism are enclosed in a sterile single use sleeve that incorporates an inflatable balloon. The balloon is about 8 cm long and is available in 36 or 48 French diameters. The ultrasound transducer and laser tip are movable (axially and radially) within the inflated balloon, which is fixed within the lumen of the prostate (Fig. 3). After the balloon has been inflated with water and maintained at 2 atm, the irregular lumen of the prostatic urethra is reconfigured into a round cylinder. Superficial blood vessels are compressed, and a smooth nonbloody surface for optimal laser irradiation is formed.

The ultrasound transducer and laser tip are controlled axially by a handle that, when squeezed, pulls the transducer and laser prism back at an operator-controlled rate. The radial position of the tip is controlled by a rotating mechanism that has stops at each position along the hours of the clock (Fig. 4). The device also comes with a disinfection system, a power meter, and an ultrasound phantom to test the integrity and operation of these systems before patient use.

This device was initially tested on a series of canine prostate glands. Two separate studies (Assimos et al. 1991; Roth and Aretz 1991) were conducted at the Lahey Clinic Medical Center and at Bowman-Gray School of Medicine. In the hyperplastic canine prostate gland, these studies showed that Nd:YAG laser irradiation at 20–50 W and a pull rate of 1 mm/s could result in removal of substantial amounts of prostatic tissue. No clinically significant bleeding and no postoperative obstruction from passage of tissue occurred in these animals. Characteristically, the depth of penetration was approximately 1 cm on either side of the balloon. Necrosed tissue sloughed over a 3–4 week period, with complete healing and reepithelial-

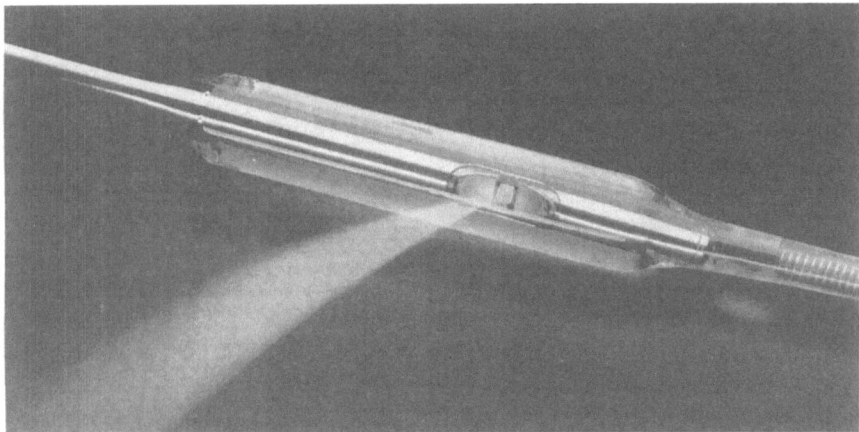

Fig. 3. Inflated 48 French balloon. Laser light and ultrasound beam penetrate balloon into tissue. (From Roth and Aretz 1991)

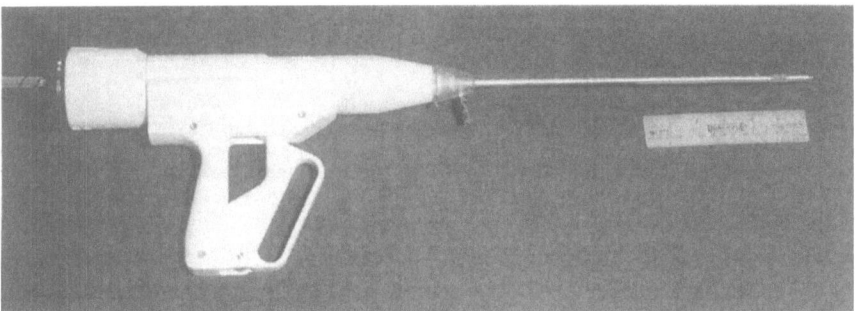

Fig. 4. Handle mechanism controls axial position of laser and ultrasound and also pull rate. By rotating back ring, radial position of tip is controlled

ization at about 6 weeks. The prostatic fossa when healed showed almost complete hollowing out and a defect comparable to that seen with conventional transurethral resection (Fig. 5). The outcome of these animal studies prompted the initiation of human clinical studies.

Human Clinical Studies

A human clinical study was initiated in November 1990 at the Lahey Clinic Medical Center and at Boston University School of Medicine. Shortly thereafter, this study was expanded to other sites in the United States, Europe, and Japan. An initial

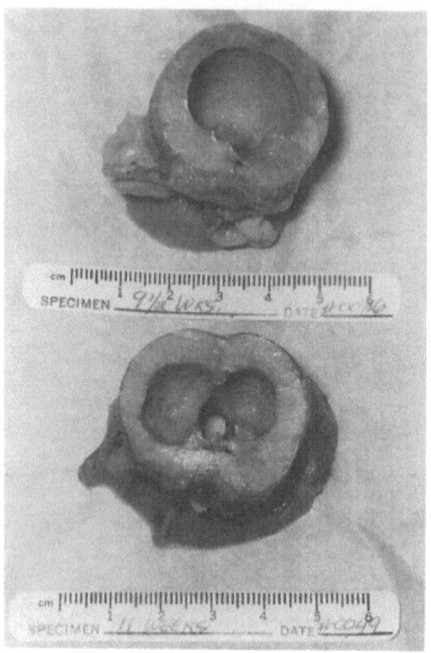

Fig. 5. Top, Fixed cross section of 30 g canine prostate harvested at 9.5 weeks after five laser lesions had been created at 20–25 W. Complete removal of interior of prostate. Bottom, Fixed cross section of canine prostate harvested at 11 weeks after two 20 W passes on the right side and two 40 W passes on the left side. (From Roth and Aretz 1991)

United States protocol[1] approved by the Food and Drug Administration (FDA) was designed to test the efficacy of the TULIP procedure in patients with documented symptomatic benign prostatic hyperplasia (BPH). As with any procedure that does not provide a specimen for pathologic examination, patients were carefully screened to rule out carcinoma of the prostate gland with tests of prostate-specific antigen, digital rectal examination, transrectal ultrasonography, and transrectal biopsy, when indicated. Only patients who had documented symptomatic BPH, a prostate gland of less than 75 ml in volume, a peak uroflow of less than 15 ml/s, and a measured residual volume of greater than 30 ml were entered into the study. Treatment outcome was measured by comparing each patient's changes in peak urinary flow and symptoms scores from preoperative values with changes at 3 weeks, 6 weeks, 3 months, 6 months, and 12 months in which efficacy end-points are recognized

[1] Investigators included R. Roth, Lahey Clinic Medical Center; R. Babayan, Boston University School of Medicine; D. McCullough, Bowman-Gray School of Medicine, J. Gordon, North Mississippi Medical Center; J. Reese, Stanford University; E. Crawford, University of Colorado; H. Fuselier, Ochsner Clinic; R. Murchison, Fort Worth, TX; K. Kaye, Abbott Northwestern Hospital, Minneapolis, MN; and J. Smith, Vanderbilt University, Nashville, TN.

by the American Urological Association cooperative benign prostatic hyperplasia study and the Advisory Panel to the FDA (transcript, open public hearing; Drugs for the treatment of benign prostatic hypertrophy: efficacy and safety criteria. FDA Advisory Committee meeting, February 3, 1992). These results were also compared by means of an identical study protocol with a concomitant prospective control group of patients undergoing standard transurethral resection and with the results of several large transurethral resection studies (Bruskewitz et al. 1986; (Chilton et al. 1978; Edwards et al. 1985; Holtgrewe et al. 1989; Lepor and Rigand 1990; Mackenzie et al. 1979; Mebust et al. 1989; Nielsen et al. 1989; Roehrborn et al. 1991; Roos et al. 1989; Siroky et al. 1979).

The Procedure

For purposes of this study protocol, most patients were admitted to the hospital the morning of the procedure and discharged home after overnight observation. Methods of anesthesia included general, spinal, epidural, and intravenous sedation. Intraoperative cystoscopy just before the TULIP procedure notes the configuration of the lateral lobes and median lobe. The bladder is left filled with the cysto irrigant. For a prostate gland judged to be of small to medium size, that is, about 30 g or less, a 36 French diameter balloon is usually chosen. For a larger gland or a large median lobe, a 48 French diameter balloon is chosen. The probe is inserted into the prostatic urethra much the same way as a resectoscope sheath, and the proper initial position is determined by transrectal palpation of the small positioning marker at the distal end of the balloon, which should be located at the apex of the prostate gland. The balloon is pressurized with sterile water and maintained at 2 atm of pressure.

When the balloon is inflated, the ultrasound transducer may be activated, and an examination of the prostate gland is carried out. Critical landmarks to be identified include the bladder and bladder neck junction (Fig. 6) and the apical area (Fig. 7). These landmarks guide the start and finish positions for laser delivery. The depth of the prostate gland can be determined readily at any point within the prostatic urethra by noting periprostatic fat or capsule (Fig. 8). Additional structures, such as the prostatic vascular pedicles, vasa and seminal vesicles, and rectum, are visible for further orientation landmarks.

A typical ultrasound examination starts at the bladder neck at the 10 or 12 o'clock position and proceeds to the apex. It is repeated at the 9, 8, 7, 6, 2, 3, 4, and 5 o'clock positions. Because the known depth of laser penetration is approximately 1 cm, the laser is not directed in areas in which less than 1 cm of prostatic tissue is present. These depth variations are common and are most often seen at the junction of the prostate and bladder, at the apex of the prostate, at the 12 o'clock position, and over the rectum. When the ultrasonic anatomy of the prostate has been determined, laser treatment is begun.

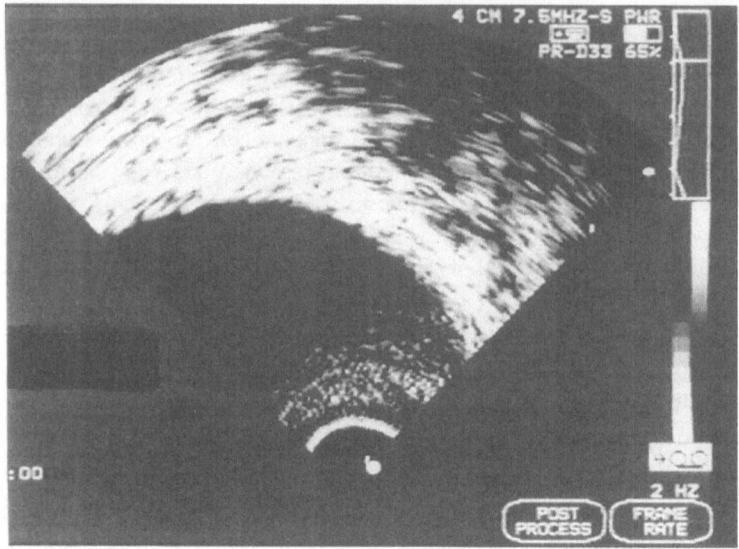

Fig. 6. TULIP ultrasound sector scan at 4 o'clock position. Intravesical prostatic tissue can be seen inside bladder

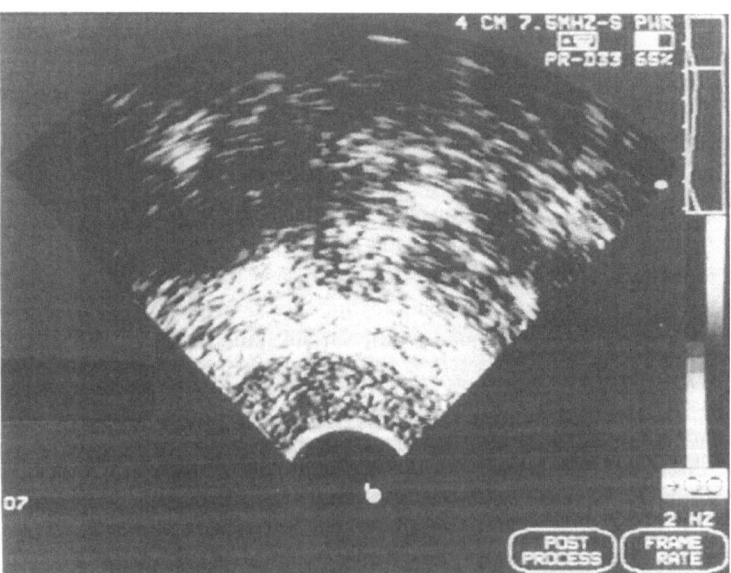

Fig. 7. Sector scan of apical prostate about 1 cm deep. This is the stop point of the laser pass

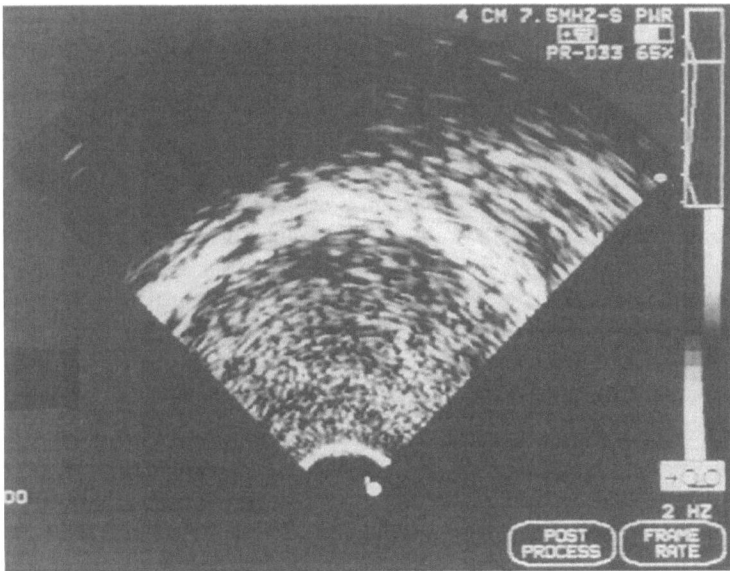

Fig. 8. Sector scan of midprostate with probe scanning 4 o'clock position. Prostate depth is 3 cm

We have empirically determined that the bladder neck requires thorough treatment, and as a result, laser delivery is begun just inside the bladder at the junction of the bladder neck and prostate where the laser beam is permitted to remain stationary for a few seconds before it is pulled as a straight line to within 1 cm of the apex. The laser dose is delivered with constant power settings in the 30–40 W range, and joules of energy delivered to a given area may be altered by squeezing the handle slower or faster than 1 mm/s, remembering that energy delivered is a product of watts times time. The typical total dose was 6000–10000 J and varied between 5000 and 20000 J. A typical pull rate is about 1 mm/s; thus, along a 3 cm prostatic urethra, each pass requires 30 s of laser time. Laser passes are placed depending on the ultrasonic anatomy but often are at the 9, 8, 7, 6, 5, 4, and 3 o'clock positions. Thus, seven laser passes at 30 s require a total of 3.5 min of laser time. In general, the average time for ultrasound examination and laser therapy is about 20 min. Median lobe obstruction requires several additional 1–2 cm separate passes directed to the median lobe. At the time of this writing, it is believed that small-to medium-size median lobes are suitable for treatment but that large mobile or pedunculated median lobes tend to be displaced to the side of the balloon and may not be well treated with the technique now used with the TULIP device.

The ultrasound picture gives information not only about where to start and stop but also about how to control laser delivery optimally. For consistent laser spot size, a standoff distance of about 4 mm from the laser prism to the balloon-urethra interface is seen and maintained. When the balloon size is incorrect, it can be seen by the ultrasound image of the balloon. Air present in the balloon or blood on the surface of the balloon can also be determined by ultrasound and corrected. In general, the net laser thermal injury cannot be well seen in real time because tissue damage develops just after the laser and ultrasound have passed through the affected tissue. For that reason, with the present device, the ultrasound transducer does not give feedback information concerning depth of tissue injury.

After laser treatment, the balloon is deflated, and the probe is removed. Bleeding is minimal, resulting simply from mechanical disruption of surface blood vessels from insertion of the balloon or probe. Laser lesions appear as depressed white lines beginning at the bladder neck and ending in the apical area. Soon thereafter, the areas between the laser lesion become hyperemic and somewhat edematous. At this point, under cystoscopic view and with the bladder distended, a percutaneous suprapubic tube, 12–14 French, is placed for postoperative drainage. A urethral catheter is not required. Patients are discharged home with the suprapubic tube in place.

Few problems are encountered during the procedure and are mainly associated with insertion of the probe. Forcing a TULIP probe through the prostate will cause bleeding. Blood between the balloon and the prostatic urethra preferentially absorbs laser energy and reduces the effectiveness of treatment. Therefore, great care should be taken in inserting the probe to avoid trauma. If an inadvertent false passage is made or a significant amount of bleeding occurs, better results will be obtained by terminating the procedure and rescheduling several days later.

Clinical Results

About 219 patients as of December 19, 1992 have been enrolled in the United States TULIP clinical study to date. A minimum of 6 months of follow-up data are available for 28 patients, with 75 patients observed to a minimum of 3 months. Patient enrollment and perioperative data for the 3 month patient cohorts for both the TULIP and transurethral resection control study groups are shown in Table 1. In the TULIP study group, hospital stay, estimated intraoperative blood

Table 1. Patient data

Factor studied	TULIP ($n = 75$)	TURP control group ($n = 18$)
Age, years mean (range)	69.1 (51–95)	65 (46–80)
Prostate size, g mean (range)	42.1 (15–101)	28.5 (20–38)
Days in hospital, mean (range)	1 (1–33)	2.8 (2–4)
Estimated blood loss, ml mean (range)	17.9 (0–200)	234 (100–400)
Operating time, min mean (range)	22.8 (5–63)	49.2 (24–85)

TULIP, transurethral ultrasound-guided laser-induced prostatectomy; TURP, transurethral resection of the prostate gland.

loss, and duration of operating times were considerably reduced compared with these same factors for the transurethral resection control group. Furthermore, this TULIP patient cohort represents the first few procedures, and therefore the learning curve, for the investigators participating in the study.

By the 3 month follow-up interval, the preoperative mean symptom score for the TULIP study group had improved from a mean 18.8 to 6.3, representing a 67.1% overall rate of improvement. These results remained constant when patients were observed to 6 months; 75% of patients undergoing the TULIP procedure had a reduction in symptom score of at least 50% and a total symptom score falling with the lower one third ("mild" symptoms) of the total possible score. Improvements in symptom scores for the TULIP study group were consistent with findings for the transurethral resection control group at these same intervals (Table 2).

Peak uroflow values for the TULIP group improved a mean 78%, with a slightly higher mean percentage improvement (124%) reported for the transurethral resection control group. Because of the wide ranges in results reported for this factor, the difference between 78% and 124% was not statistically significant (Table 3). Although peak uroflow values were improved by a minimum of 50% and improved into the "unobstructed" range for most patients in the TULIP group, patients in the transurethral resection control group were reported to have higher uroflow values at follow-up visits than patients in the TULIP group.

In the TULIP study group, 64 of 75 (85.3%) of the 3 month cohort patients met the success criteria defined in the FDA study protocol. This finding remains constant when patients are observed to 6 months; results were successful in 85.2%. Overall, the failed procedures to date resulted from inadequate laser energy delivered. Many problems appeared to resolve as experience was gained, as expertise using the ultrasound image to guide laser delivery developed, and as surgical techniques were refined by the investigator group. Six of 11 (54.5%) unsuccessful results occurred within the first 20 procedures performed. In these patients, it was common that too few laser passes were delivered overall or that laser passes were not appropriately directed according to the anatomy defined by the ultrasound image. Minor enhancements and modifications of technique have been based on these early experiences, especially with regard to treatment of intravesical or median lobe hyperplasia.

Table 2. Modified Boyarsky symptom score (Lepor and Rigaud 1990)

	TULIP	TURP control group
Preoperative mean (range)	18.8 (8–32)	17.5 (9–27)
3 months	6.3 (0–20)	6.7 (0–14)
Improvement	67.1%	64.3%
6 months	7.1 (1–19)	4.4 (0–10)
Improvement	64.7%	76%

TULIP, transurethral ultrasound-guided laser-induced prostatectomy; TURP, transurethral resection of the prostate gland.

Table 3. Peak uroflow

	TULIP	TURP control group	Literature[a]
Preoperative peak uroflow, ml/s, mean (range)	6.6 (2–14.8)	9.1 (0–14)	8–10
3 months, ml/s, mean	13 (5.1–27.8)	20.4 (5.8–49.8)	16
Improvement	78%	124%	79%–107%
6 months, ml/s, mean	12.6 (7.3–26.4)	23.2 (16–37.5)	
Improvement	75.6%	149%	

TULIP, transurethral ultrasound-guided laser-induced prostatectomy; TURP, transurethral resection of the prostate gland.
[a] References are Bruskewitz et al. 1986; Lepor and Rigaud 1990; Nielsen et al. 1989; Roehrborn et al. 1991.

Morbidity associated with the TULIP study is low (Table 4). No instance of misdirected laser energy has resulted in perforation or laser-related injury, no instance of impotence has resulted from the TULIP procedure, and no bleeding has occurred after the TULIP procedure. No patient in the TULIP group has reported

Table 4. Complications

Complication	TULIP (n = 75)	TURP control group (n = 18)	Literature[a]
Early			
Perforation	0	0	1%–18%
Blood loss	17.9 ml	234 ml	4–1150 ml
Transfusion	0	0	6%
Transurethral resection syndrome	0	0	2%
Urinary retention			
After discharge	22.7%	11%	6.5%
Fever			
Acute	2.7%	5.6%	–
Bacteriuria	28%	27.7%	1%–20%
Pain, spasm	±	±	–
Late			
Bladder neck contracture	0	8.3%	1%–6%
Urethral stricture	0	16.7%	0.5%–16.5%
Infection (3 months)	14%	0	6%–24%
Incontinence	0	0	0.2%–53%
Sexual dysfunction			
Erection	0	0	1%–20%
Retrograde ejaculation	0	50%	11%–63%

TULIP, transurethral ultrasound-guided laser-induced prostatectomy; TURP, transurethral resection of the prostate gland.
[a] References are Chilton et al. 1978; Edwards et al. 1985; Holtgrewe et al. 1989; Mackenzie et al. 1979; Mebust et al. 1989; Roos et al. 1989; Siroky et al. 1979.

episodes of retrograde ejaculation compared with a 50% incidence of this complication in the transurethral resection control group, and no patient in the TULIP group has presented with bladder neck contracture compared with the 8.3% rate of occurrence in the transurethral resection control group. These findings may also shed light on why peak uroflow values are lower after the TULIP procedure than after transurethral resection. Scarring or damage to the bladder neck after electrosurgical resection, which compromises the function of the sphincter but permits a higher peak flow rate to be attained, appears to be avoided by the TULIP procedure. Early complications in the TULIP group show a higher incidence of postoperative urinary retention than is found after transurethral resection. This finding reflects the differences in the modes of tissue removal for the two procedures. As was discussed earlier, necrosed tissue is passed over time during the early postoperative period after the TULIP procedure, and until postoperative edema subsides and sufficient tissue has sloughed to relieve outlet obstruction, suprapubic tubes are left in place.

Postoperative Care

Most patients require minimal postoperative pain medication. Postoperative medications usually include a urinary antiseptic for 2 or 3 weeks, and a nonsteroidal anti-inflammatory agent is commonly prescribed before and after the operation for 1 week to reduce edema and inflammation. Occasionally, a patient may complain of bladder spasm, and antispasmodics can be prescribed. No significant bleeding occurs postoperatively, and irrigations are unnecessary. Because no irrigation is used during or after the TULIP procedure, complications from hypervolemia and electrolyte imbalance do not occur. Although patients were hospitalized overnight for these clinical studies, postoperative events requiring overnight hospitalization were rare, and it is possible that the TULIP procedure could be performed on an outpatient basis.

Postoperative Course

Most patients experience some degree of acute obstruction after the TULIP procedure because of swelling and edema of the prostatic urethra. The suprapubic tube enables the patient to determine when the obstruction has resolved and when the tube can be removed. Because the TULIP procedure does not instantaneously remove prostatic tissue as does traditional transurethral resection of the prostate, it is necessary for the treated tissue to become necrotic and to slough out before normal voiding occurs. This process usually takes between 5 and 21 days. After about

5–7 days, the patient is instructed to close the valve on the suprapubic tube and to try to void. When the patient states he can void adequately and comfortably, he returns for an office visit to remove the suprapubic tube. Rarely do pieces of tissues occlude the suprapubic tube, and no instances of urethral occlusion have occurred from sloughed tissue. Tissue usually passes as fine white debris. In the typical postoperative course, urinary flow increases and symptoms decrease between 2 and 3 weeks after the procedure, and improvement continues to about the 3 month period. From that point on, results usually remain stable.

Comment

Preliminary results of this clinical study show that Nd:YAG laser energy delivered through the TULIP system is capable of safely removing substantial amounts of prostatic tissue and the TULIP procedure has certain advantages compared with transurethral resection of the prostate. Early results from the TULIP procedure are comparable to results from a controlled transurethral resection group and to historical transurethral resection data in the literature (Bruskewitz et al. 1986; Chilton et al. 1978; Edwards et al. 1985; Holtgrewe et al. 1989; Lepor and Rigaud 1990; Mackenzie et al. 1979; Mebust et al. 1989; Nielsen et al. 1989; Roehrborn et al. 1991; Roos et al. 1989; Siroky et al. 1979) (Figs. 9 and 10). The advantages of the TULIP procedure vs standard transurethral resection are shorter hospitalization, significantly reduced bleeding, no irrigant-related complications, reduced incidences of bladder neck contracture and stricture, and a substantial reduction in the occurrence of retrograde ejaculation. With proper training, the learning curve appears to be three to five patients. The disadvantages of the TULIP procedure at this stage of development are the need for prolonged catheterization by suprapubic tube, difficulties in treating large median lobe obstruction, insufficient data regarding treatment of a large prostate gland more than 75 g, and the lack of real-time ultrasound feedback for precise adjustment of the laser dose. Nevertheless,

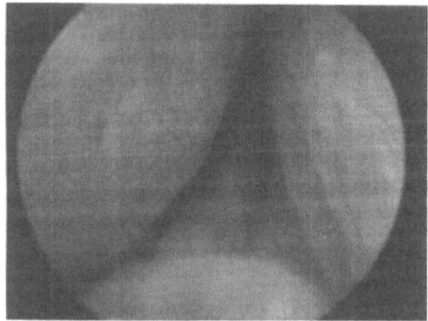

Fig. 9. Preoperative view of 30 g human prostate gland showing trilobar obstruction. Peak uroflow was about 5 ml/s, and modified Boyarsky symptom score was 22

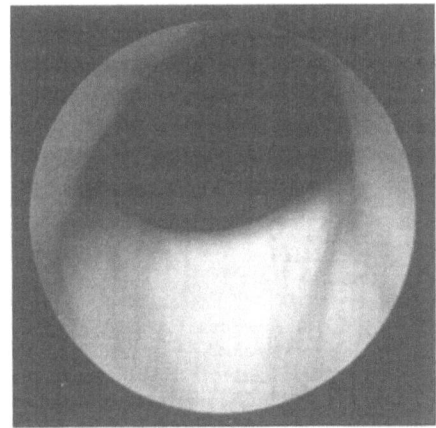

Fig. 10. Video result 6 months after TULIP procedure in same patient as seen in Fig. 9. Peak uroflow was 22 ml/s, and modified Boyarsky symptom score was 1-2. Widely patent prostatic urethra with normal antegrade ejaculation

the advantages of the TULIP procedure may make it competitive with traditional transurethral resection. Further advances in ultrasound and laser technology may overcome these deficiencies and result in a procedure that may even surpass the outcome of conventional transurethral resection of the prostate.

References

Assimos DG, McCullough DL, Woodruff RD, Harrison LH, Hart LJ, Li W-J (1991) Canine transurethral laser-induced prostatectomy. J Endourol 5:145-149

Beisland HO, Sander S (1986) First clinical experiences on neodymium-YAG laser irradiation of localized prostatic cancer. Scand J Urol Nephrol 20:113-117

Bruskewitz RC, Larsen EH, Madsen PO, Dørflinger T (1986) 3-Year followup of urinary symptoms after transurethral resection of the prostate. J Urol 136:613-615

Chilton CP, Morgan RJ, England HR, Paris AMI, Blandy JP (1978) A critical evaluation of the results of transurethral resection of the prostate. Br J Urol 50:542-546

Cohen MS, Warner RS (1988) Treatment of bladder neck obstruction utilizing the neodymium:YAG laser. Abstract. Lasers Surg Med 8:170

Costello AJ, Johnson DE (1991) Nd:YAG laser ablation of the prostate as a treatment for benign prostatic hypertrophy. Abstract. J Endourol 5 [Suppl 1]:S128

Edwards LE, Bucknall TE, Pittam MR, Richardson DR, Stanek J (1985) Transurethral resection of the prostate and bladder neck incision: a review of 700 cases. Br J Urol 57:168-171

Fisher JC (1987) Basic laser physics and interaction of laser light with soft tissue. In: Shapshay SM (ed) Endoscopic laser surgery handbook. Dekker, New York, pp 1-130

Frank F (1988) Noncontact delivery systems and accessories for the application of the Nd:YAG laser in endoscopy and surgery. In: Joffe SN, Oguro Y (eds) Advances in Nd:YAG laser surgery. Springer, Berlin Heidelberg New York, pp 10-18

Hofstetter A (1986) Lasers in urology. Lasers Surg Med 6:412-414

Holtgrewe HL, Mebust WK, Dowd JB, Cockett ATK, Peters PC, Proctor C (1989) Transurethral prosta-tectomy: Practice aspects of the dominant operation in American urology. J Urol 141:248–253

Johnson DE, Levinson AK, Greskovich FJ, Cromeens DM, Ro JY, Costello AJ, Wishnow KI (1991a) Transurethral laser prostatectomy using a right-angle laser delivery system. In: Watson GM, Steiner RW, Pietrasitta JJ (eds) Lasers in urology, laparoscopy, and general surgery. Proc Spie 1421:36–41

Johnson DE, Costello AJ, Wishnow KI (1991b) Transurethral laser prostatectomy using a right angle laser delivery system (abstract). Lasers Surg Med 11 [Suppl 3]:76

Lepor H, Rigaud G (1990) The efficacy of transurethral resection of the prostate in men with moderate symptoms of prostatism. J Urol 143:533–537

Mackenzie AR, Levine N, Scheinman HZ (1979) Operative blood loss in transurethral prostatectomy. J Urol 122:47–48

McNicholas T (1988) Endoscopic application of lasers in urology. Br J Hosp Med 40:197–206

Mebust WK, Holtgrewe HL, Cockett ATK, Peters PC, and Writing Committee (1989) Transurethral prostatectomy: immediate and postoperative complications. A cooperative study of 13 participating institutions evaluating 3,885 patients. J Urol 141:243–247

Newman C, Jacques SL (1991) Laser penetration into prostate for various wavelengths (abstract). Lasers Surg Med 11 [Suppl 3]:75–76

Nielsen KT, Christensen MM, Madsen PO, Bruskewitz RC (1989) Symptom analysis and uroflowmetry 7 years after transurethral resection of the prostate. J Urol 142:1251–1253

Roehrborn CG, McConnell JD, Eddy DM (1991) Outcome analysis after treatment for benign prostatic hyperplasia (BPH) by various modalities: a confidence profile analysis (abstract). J Urol 145:364A

Roos NP, Wennberg JE, Malenka DJ, Fisher ES, McPherson K, Anderson TF, Cohen MM, Ramsey E (1989) Mortality and reoperation after open and transurethral resection of the prostate for benign prostatic hyperplasia. N Engl J Med 320:1120–1124

Roth RA, Aretz HT (1991) Transurethral ultrasound-guided laser-induced prostatectomy (TULIP procedure): a canine prostate feasibility study. J Urol 146:1128–1135

Roth RA, Aretz HT, Lage A (1990) Poster presented at the American Urological Association annual meeting, New Orleans, Louisiana, 13–16 May 1990

Shanberg AM, Tansey LA, Baghdassarian R (1985) The use of the neodymium YAG laser in prosta-totómy (abstract). J Urol 133:196A

Silber N, Servadio C (1991) Postprostatectomy bladder neck obstruction cleared by Nd:YAG. Urol Times 19:12

Siroky MB, Olsson CA, Krane RJ (1979) The flow rate nomogram: I. Development. J Urol 122:665–668

α-Adrenergic Blockade in the Treatment of Benign Prostatic Hyperplasia

F.C.Lowe and H.Lepor

Introduction

Benign prostatic hyperplasia (BPH) is the most common neoplasm in men; it develops with increasing age and is a spectrum of both glandular and stromal hyperplasia. The stroma contains a substantial amount of smooth muscle (Bartsch et al. 1979). Morphometrically, men with symptomatic BPH are more likely to have a greater proportion of stromal hyperplasia (Shapiro et al. 1992). Since the symptoms of prostatism are the major indication for prostatectomy, medications and techniques that relieve symptoms without surgery have been actively investigated. α-Adrenergic antagonists which decrease the tension of prostatic smooth muscle are such agents. This chapter will outline both the laboratory and clinical experiences with these agents for the treatment of BPH.

Rationale for α-Blockade

Marco Caine proposed that infravesical obstruction in men with symptomatic BPH is comprised of both static and dynamic components (Caine 1986). The dynamic component of obstruction is determined primarily by the tone of the prostate smooth muscle; the static component of obstruction is related primarily to the mechanical obstruction caused by the enlarged prostate adenoma. Given the dynamic factors for prostatic obstruction, pharmacologic strategies for the treatment of BPH have been directed towards relaxing the prostate smooth muscle. The tone of the prostate smooth muscle is mediated by the autonomic nervous system. Therefore, pharmacologic agents interfering with the release, degradation, or action of the neurotransmitters mediating prostate smooth muscle tone should favorably alter resistance to urinary outflow in the prostatic urethra.

Raz and associates observed in 1973 that the rat prostate contracted in the presence of norepinephrine (Raz et al. 1973). Caine and associates subsequently demonstrated that human prostate adenoma and capsule also contracted in the presence of norepinephrine (Caine et al. 1975). Norepinephrine is the neurotransmitter released by postganglionic adrenergic neurons. Radioligand receptor binding studies have shown that the human prostate contains α_1 and α_2-adrenoceptors (Gup et al. 1990). In vitro isometric tension studies have demonstrated that the contractile properties of human prostate adenomas are mediated primarily by α_1-adrenoceptors (Gup et al. 1989). Specifically, the contractile response of prostate adenomas to α_1-adrenergic, α_2-adrenergic, and muscarinic cholinergic agonists have been evaluated using the selective agonists phenylephrine, UK 14, 304, and carbachol, respectively (Lepor et al. 1988). The magnitude of the contractile response (gram tension per gram tissue) to phenylephrine was tenfold and sixfold greater than that observed for UK 14, 304, and carbachol, respectively (Lepor et al. 1988). Based upon the afore-mentioned physiological and pharmacological observations, α-adrenergic antagonists appear to decrease the resistance along the prostatic urethra by relaxing the smooth muscle component of the prostate. Comparative binding and functional studies of lower genitourinary tissues demonstrated that α_1-adrenoceptors are sparse in the bladder body and abundant in the bladder base and prostate (Shapiro and Lepor 1987). Thus, α-adrenergic antagonists are ideally suited for the treatment of bladder outlet obstruction since the resistance along the bladder outlet can be selectively reduced without impairing detrusor contractility.

Clinical Experiences Using α-Blockade

Since Marco Caine reported in 1976 that α-blockers are effective for the treatment of BPH (Caine et al. 1976), at least 20 clinical trial evaluating α-blockers for the treatment of BPH have been reported (Table 1). The majority of these studies were deficient in their study designs. The criteria for enrollment, assessment of efficacy, and statistical analyses were not standardized. Only five studies enrolled greater than 30 patients into treatment arms. The duration of treatment exceeded 2 months in five studies. Fifteen clinical trials were randomized and placebo controlled. Assessment of efficacy was based upon uroflowmetry and quantitative symptom score assessments in 19 and four studies, respectively. Phenoxybenzamine, nicer-goline, thymoxamine, prazosin, alfuzosin, terazosin, and YM12617 are α-blockers that have been evaluated for the treatment of symptomatic BPH (Table 2). Of the 20 reported clinical trials, 18 confirmed Caine's original observation that α-blockers are effective for the treatment of BPH. A comprehensive review of all the reported clinical studies is beyond the scope of this chapter. A representative randomized, placebo-controlled, clinical trial of phenoxybenzamine (Caine et al. 1978) and prazosin (Kirby et al. 1987) for the treatment of BPH are reviewed in order to illustrate the efficacy and toxicity of these agents. In addition, in-depth review of the multicenter, randomized, placebo-controlled double-blind study of terazosin (Hytrin) will be presented (Lepor et al. 1992).

Phenoxybenzamine

Caine and associates reported on a placebo-controlled, double-blind study of the effect of phenoxybenzamine on benign prostatic obstruction (Caine et al.

Table 1. Study designs for α-blockers in BPH

	Patients	Follow-up	Randomized placebo	Assessment of efficacy	
	(#n)	(weeks)		Uroflowmetry	Symptom score
Phenoxybenzamine					
Gerstenberg et al. 1980	9	4	No	Yes	No
Caine et al. 1978	24	2	Yes	Yes	No
Boreham et al. 1977	30	1	No	No	No
Ferrie and Pate. 1987	21	5	Yes	Yes	No
Brooks et al. 1983	10	4	Yes	Yes	No
Abrams et al. 1982	21	4	Yes	Yes	No
Thymoxamine					
Giberti et al. 1984	8	1	Yes	Yes	No
Nicergoline					
Ronchi et al. 1982	16	1/2	Yes	Yes	No
Prazosin					
Martorana et al. 1984	9	2	Yes	Yes	No
Hedlund et al. 1983	20	4	Yes	Yes	No
Kirby et al. 1987	28	4	Yes	Yes	No
Chapple et al. 1990	46	12	Yes	Yes	No
Alfuzosin					
Tacovou et al. 1987	11	8	Yes	Yes	No
Ramsay et al. 1985	20	12	Yes	Yes	No
Indorman					
Scott and Abrams 1989	18	4	Yes	Yes	No
YM12617					
Kawabe and Nijima 1988	77	2	No	Yes	No
Terazosin					
Dunzendorfer 1988	15	4	No	Yes	Yes
Lepor et al. 1990	45	30	No	Yes	Yes
Fabricias et al. 1990	53	24	Yes	Yes	Yes
Lepor et al. 1992	264	16	Yes	Yes	Yes

1978). There were 50 patients with BPH who were randomized to receive phenoxybenzamine 10 mg or placebo b.i.d. The clinical trial was only 14 days in duration, and 49 patients completed the trial. The assessment of efficacy was based on improvement in urinary flow rates and frequency of micturition. The peak urinary flow rates in the phenoxybenzamine and placebo groups improved 82% and 30%, respectively. There was a significantly greater improvement in day- and night-time urinary frequency among phenoxybenzamine-treated patients. The primary limitation of phenoxybenzamine was the incidence and severity of adverse reactions. Eleven patients experienced tiredness, dizziness, impaired ejaculation,

Table 2. α-Blockers

Nonselective α-blockers
  Phenoxybenzamine
  Thymoxamine

Selective alpha blockers
  Prazosin
  Nicergoline
  Alfuzosin
  YM-12617

Selective long-acting α_1-blockers
  Terazosin
  Doxazosin

nasal stuffiness, or difficulty with visual accommodation. A single adverse reaction was observed in the placebo group.

Prazosin

Kirby and associates reported on a randomized, placebo-controlled study evaluating prazosin for the treatment of prostatic obstruction (Kirby et al. 1987). A total of 80 men age 50–80 years with BPH were randomized to receive 2 mg of prazosin b.i.d. or placebo. Only 55 patients completed the 1 month clinical trial. Assessment of efficacy was based on improvement in urinary flow rates, frequency of micturition, and postvoid residual volume. The peak urinary flow rate improved 59% and 6% in the prazosin- and placebo-treated groups, respectively. The observed improvement in residual urine and voiding frequency in the prazosin-treated group were statistically significant. No adverse reactions were observed in the prazosin-treated group, whereas two patients in the placebo-treated group complained of dizziness and diarrhea. Orthostatic hypotension and erectile or ejaculatory dysfunction were not observed in either the placebo- or prazosin-treated groups.

Terazosin

A total of 487 patients were enrolled into the large, multicenter, Phase III, double-blind, parallel group, placebo-controlled study of once-a-day administration of terazosin to patients with symptomatic BPH (Lepor et al. 1992). The study was divided into two parts: (1) a 4 week, single-blind, placebo lead-in period and (2) a 12 week double-blind treatment period (Fig. 1). The screening procedures included a complete medical history, thorough physical examination, and a complete urological examination (urinalysis, urine culture, renal imaging study, and prostate ultrasound were completed during the placebo lead-in period). The body weight, blood pressure, and pulse rate were measured, and adverse events were recorded at each study visit. The peak and mean urinary flow rates and Boyarsky symptom scores were also evaluated at each study visit. The Boyarsky symptom questionnaire

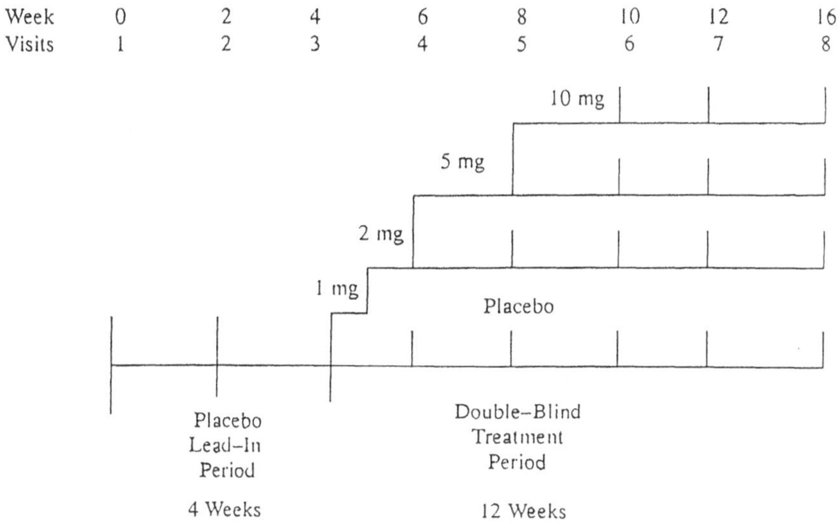

Week	0	2	4	6	8	10	12	16
Visits	1	2	3	4	5	6	7	8

Fig. 1. Terazosin BPH multicenter fixed-dose study

scored the frequency and severity of nine urinary symptoms associated with BPH on a numerical scale of 0–3, with zero indicating the absence of symptoms and three denoting severe symptoms (Boyarsky et al. 1977). The summation of the obstruction (hesitancy, intermittency, terminal dribbling, force of stream, and sensation of incomplete emptying) and irritative (nocturia, daytime frequency, urgency, and dysuria) symptoms yields the obstructive score and irritative score, respectively.

There were 314 patients who entered the double-blind treatment period following the placebo lead-in period provided: (1) all selection criteria were satisfied; (2) a symptom score was ≥1 on at least two of the symptoms classified as obstructive; (3) the peak urinary flow rate was at least 5 ml/s but not more than 12 ml/s at each visit of the placebo lead-in period and the voided volume was at least 150 ml; and (4) the residual volume obtained by catheterization was less than or equal to 200 ml. At the final visit of the placebo lead-in period, qualifying patients were assigned to double-blind treatment with placebo, 2, 5, or 10 mg of terazosin once daily. All patients assigned to the terazosin treatment groups were given 1 mg of terazosin on the first 3 days of double-blind treatment followed by 2 mg of terazosin for 11 days. Those patients assigned to the 2 mg terazosin dose continued to receive 2 mg of terazosin for the remainder of the study while those patients assigned to the 5 or 10 mg terazosin dosage groups received 5 mg of terazosin of the next 2 weeks. Those patients assigned to the 5 mg terazosin group then continued to receive 5 mg of terazosin for the remainder of the study while those assigned to the 10 mg terazosin dosage group received 10 mg of terazosin or the remaining 8 weeks (Fig. 1).

Of the 314 patients randomized, 264 (84%) completed the 12 week double-blind treatment. The distribution of indications for patient withdrawals during treatment was similar for the four treatment groups, with administrative reasons being the predominant cause. All treatment groups were comparable in regards to all parameters assessed.

The Boyarsky symptom questionnaire was used as the primary measure of symptomatic improvement. There were statistically significant (p <0.05) decreases from baseline in obstructive, irritative, and total symptom scores for all terazosin treatment groups (Table 3). All terazosin treatment groups had significantly greater decreases in irritative and total scores than the placebo group. The decreases in obstructive score for the 5 and 10 mg terazosin treatment groups were also significantly greater than for the placebo group. The improvement in symptom scores was dose related. The change in total symptom scores was summarized according to the percentage of patients experiencing >30%–50% improvement (improved) and >50% improvement (markedly improved). The percentage of patients experiencing >30% improvement in the total symptom scores for the placebo, 2, 5, and 10 mg treatment groups was 38%, 54%, 63%, and 70%, respectively. The percentage of patients experiencing greater than 30% improvement in total symptom score in the 5 and 10 mg treatment groups was significantly greater than in the placebo group. The improvement in total symptom score plateaued at maintenance week 2 (week 6) for the 10 mg treatment group. The relationship between symptom score and time suggests that the effect of α-blockade with terazosin occurs within 2 weeks.

A statistically significant improvement from baseline was observed in the peak and mean urinary flow rates for all treatment groups, including placebo. The 10 mg treatment group had significantly larger increases from baseline in peak and mean urinary flow rates than the placebo group. The 5 mg treatment group also had a significantly larger increase in mean flow rate than the placebo group. The relationship between change in urinary flow rate and maintenance dose suggests a dose related response. The categorical breakdown of change in peak urinary flow rate is summarized for each of the treatment groups (Table 4). The percentages of patients experiencing >30% increase in peak urinary flow rate in the placebo, 2, 5, and 10 mg treatment groups were 25%, 36%, 35%, and 58%, respectively. A significantly greater proportion of patients in the 10 mg terazosin treatment groups experienced an improvement of this magnitude than in the placebo group.

Table 3. Multicenter terazosin study: categorical breakdown of total symptom scores (from Lepor et al. 1992)

	Deteriorated >10%	Within 10% of baseline	Improved >10%–30%	Improved >30%–50%	Improved >50%
Placebo	8 (13%)	17 (28%)	12 (20%)	14 (23%)	9 (15%)
2 mg	7 (10%)	4 (6%)	20 (29%)	20 (29%)	17 (25%)
5 mg	1 (2%)	5 (8%)	18 (28%)	23 (35%)	18 (28%)
10 mg	2 (3%)	2 (3%)	14 (24%)	21 (36%)	20 (34%)

Comparisons of proportions responding (>30% improvement; against placebo): 2 mg, $p = 0.054$; 5 mg, $p = 0.004$; 10 mg, $p = 0.001$.

Table 4. Multicenter terazosin study: evaluable patients categorized by change from baseline in unadjusted peak flow rate (from Lepor et al. 1992)

Treatment group	Total(n)	$< -10\%$	$-10\% - 10\%$	$11\% - 30\%$	$>30\%$
Placebo	58	6 (10%)	22 (38%)	15 (26%)	15 (26%)
2 mg	64	7 (11%)	17 (27%)	16 (25%)	24 (38%)
5 mg	65	4 (6%)	19 (29%)	19 (29%)	23 (35%)
10 mg	57	2 (4%)	10 (18%)	11 (19%)	34 (60%)

Table 5. Multicenter terazosin study: selected adverse events (from Lepor et al. 1992)

	Placebo	2 mg	5 mg	10 mg
Asthenia	2 (2.6%)	5 (6.2%)	5 (6.4%)	8 (10.1%)
Flu Syndrome	1 (1.3%)	1 (1.2%)	3 (3.8%)	5 (6.3%)
Headache	5 (6.6%)	5 (6.2%)	1 (1.3%)	4 (5.1%)
Postural hypotension	0	2 (2.5%)	6 (7.7%)	4 (5.1%)
Dizziness	2 (2.6%)	5 (6.2%)	3 (3.8%)	9 (11.4%)
Urinary tract infection	0	0	0	3 (3.8%)

Overall, the adverse events in the four treatment groups were minor and reversible (Table 5). Although higher frequencies of asthenia, flu syndrome, and dizziness were observed in the terazosin treatment groups, the differences from placebo were not statistically significant when tested using Fisher's exact test. One patients in the 10 mg treatment group developed syncope at the 5 mg dose of terazosin. The incidence of syncope in the 10 mg treatment group was thus 1/79 (1.3%); the incidence of syncope for all terazosin treated patients was $<0.5\%$.

Vital signs (blood pressure and pulse) were essentially unchanged. Although larger decreases in systolic blood pressure were observed in the 5 mg and 10 mg groups, the differences among groups was not significant. The 5 mg and 10 mg terazosin groups had significantly larger decreases in diastolic blood pressure than the placebo group.

Summary

Adverse Events

One of the primary concerns regarding the management of BPH with α_1-blockade has been that elderly patients would not tolerate the adverse events associated with drug therapy, particularly syncope and orthostatic hypotension. The proportion of patients withdrawn from the multicenter study during the double-blind treatment owing to adverse events was similar for the terazosin and placebo groups. The between group comparisons demonstrated that the mean decrease in diastolic blood pressure was significantly greater in the 5 and 10 mg terazosin treatment groups than in the placebo group, whereas the change in systolic blood pressure did not differ significantly from placebo. The changes in diastolic blood pressure was not clinically significant. The adverse events previously associated with terazosin administration for the management of hypertension include postural hypotension, asthenia, dizziness, headache and somnolence (Rudd 1986). Although higher frequencies of asthenia and dizziness were observed in terazosin treatment groups, the differences from placebo were not significant (Lepor et al. 1992). All adverse events were reversible upon discontinuing the drug. Evening administration of the long-acting α_1-blocker decreases incidence of asthenia and dizziness (Lepor et al. 1990).

Symptoms

The improvement in obstruction, irritative, and total symptom scores relative to baseline values was significant for all treatment arms in the multicenter study. Obstructive symptoms in particular improved dramatically, between 40%–55% for terazosin treated patients. The placebo effect of a "drug" on the symptoms of prostatism (Isaacs 1990) has been confirmed. The improvement in symptom scores appears to be dose related. The improvements in symptom scores did not plateau within the dose ranges evaluated in the multicenter study suggesting that further efficacy may be achieved by doses exceeding 10 mg.

Flow Rates

A significant improvement in peak and mean urinary flow rates relative to baseline has been observed for all dosages of terazosin. Approximately 50% improvement will be observed. The 10 mg dosage caused larger increases than lower dosages. The improvements in urinary flow rates are dose related; further efficacy may be achieved with doses exceeding 10 mg.

Predictors of Response

No clinical or urodynamic parameter has been identified that will be predictive of a clinical response to selective α_1-blockade. Analysis of response over time suggests that the clinical response to an α-blocker plateaus within 2 weeks at a particular dose level. Thus, it is reasonable to titrate all potential candidates to 10 mg of terazosin providing limiting adverse events do not occur rather than conducting expensive, invasive, and urodynamic studies.

Conclusions

Although the protocol designs for evaluating α-blockers in BPH have been highly variable, the improvement observed for urinary flow rates has been highly consistent. Overall, urinary flow rates improve approximately 50% following administration of α-blockers. The degree of symptomatic improvement following administration of the various α-blockers is equivocal since quantitative symptom score questionnaires have rarely been utilized to assess this fundamental outcomes parameter. The toxicity associates with the α-blockers has been highly variable. The incidence and severity of adverse reactions associated with the nonselective α-blockers, such as phenoxybenzamine, are far greater than the toxicity of selective α-blockers such as prazosin and terazosin. The implication of the clinical experience with α-blockers for BPH is that efficacy is dependent upon α_1-adrenoceptor blockade, whereas toxicity is related to α_2-adrenoceptor blockade.

The short-term efficacy and safety of once-a-day, long-acting, selective, α_1-blockers in the treatment of symptomatic BPH has been confirmed. The role of α-blockade in the long-term management of BPH has yet to defined. Morphometric analysis of prostatic stromal content might identify the group of patients who will have the best long-term responses.

References

Abrams PH, Shah PJR, Stone R et al. (1982) Baldder outflow obstruction treated with phenoxybenzamine. Br J Urol 54:527–530

Bartsch G, Mueller HR, Oberholzer M, Rohr HP (1979) Light microscopic stereological analysis of the normal human prostate and of benign prosttic hyperplasia. J Urol 122:487–491

Boreham PF, Braithwaite P, Milewski P et al. (1977) Alpha adrenergic blockers in prostatism. Br J Surg 64:756–757

Boyarsky S, Jones G, Paulson DF et al. (1977) A new look at bladder neck obstruction by the Food and Drug Administration regulators: guidelines for investigation of benign prostatic hypertrophy. Trans Am Ass Genito Urin Surg 68:29–31

Brooks ME, Sidi AA, Hanani Y et al. (1983) Ineffectiveness of phenoxybenzamine in treatment of benign prostatic hyperptrophy: a controlled study. Urology 21:474–478

Caine M (1986) The present role of alpha-adrenergic blockers in the treatment of benign prostatic hyperthrophy. J Urol 136:1

Caine M, Raz S, Ziegler M (1975) Adrenergic and cholinergic receptors in the human prostate, prostatic capsule, and bladder neck. Br J Urol 47:193

Caine M, Pfau A, Perlberg S (1976) The use of alpha adrenergic blockers in benign prostatic obstruction. Br J Urol 48:255–263

Caine M, Perlberg S, Meretyk S (1978) A placebo-controlled double-blind study of the effect of phenoxybenzamine in benign prostatic obstruction. Br J Urol 50:551–554

Chapple CR, Christmas TJ, Milroy EJG (1990) A twelve-week placebo controlled study of prazosin in the treatment of prostatic obstruction. Urol Int 45 [Suppl]: 47–55

Dunzendorfer U (1988) Clinial experience: symptomatic management of BPH with terazosin. Urology 32:27–31

Fabricias PG, Weizert P, Dunzendorfer V et al. (1990) Efficacy of once-a-day terazosin in bening prostatic hyperplasia. Prostate Suppl 3:85–93

Ferrie BG, Patersson PJ (1987) Phenoxybenzamine in prostatic hypertrophy. A double-blind study. Br J Urol 59:63–75

Gerstenberg T, Blaabjerg J, Lykkegaard N et al. (1980) Phenoxybenzamine reduces bladder outlet obstruction in benign prostatic hyperplasia: a urodynamic investigation. Invest Urol 18:29–31

Giberti C, Damonte P, Michelott P et al. (1984) The effect of thymoxamine in benign prostatic hypertrophy: a double-blind crossover study. IRCS Med Sci 12:591

Gup DI, Shapiro E, Baumann M et al. (1989) The contractile properties of human prostate adenomas are unrelated to the development of infravesical obstruction. Prostate 15:105–114

Gup DI, Shapiro E, Baumann M et al. (1990) Autonomic receptors in asymptomatic and symptomatic BPH. J Urol 143:179–185

Hedlund H, Anderson KE, Ek A (1983) Effects of prazosin in patients with benign prostatic obstruction. J Urol 130:275–278

Iacovou JW, Dunn M (1987) Indoramin an effective new drug in the management of bladder outflow obstruction. Br J Urol 60:526–528

Isaacs JT (1990) Importance of natural history of BPH in the evaluation of pharmacologic intervention. Prostate Suppl 3:9–26

Kawabe K, Niijima T (1987) Use of an alpha$_1$ blockers, YM-12617, in micturition difficulty. Urol Int 42:280–284

Kirby RS, Coppinger SWC, Corcoran MO, et al. (1987) Prazosin in the treatment of prostatic obstruction: a placebo-controlled study. Br J Urol 60:136–142

Lepor H, Gup DI, Baumann M, Shapiro E (1988) Laboratory assessment of terazosin and alpha$_1$ blockade in prostatic hyperplasia. Urology [Suppl] 32:21–26

Lepor H, Knapp-Maloney G, Sunshine H (1990) An open label dose titration study evaluation terazosin for the treatment of symptomatic BPH. J Urol 144:1263–1266

Lepor H, Auerbach S, Drago J et al. (1992) A randomized, placebo-controlled multicenter study of the efficacy and safety of terazosin in the treatment of benign prostatic hyperplasia. J Urol 148:1467–1474

Martorana G, Giberti C, Damonte P et al. (1984) The effect of prazosin in benign prostatic hypertrophy, a placebo controlled double-blind study. IRCS Med Sci 12:11–12

Ramsay JWA, Scott GI, Whitfield N (1985) A double-blind controlled trial of a new alpha$_1$ blocking drug in the treatment of bladder outflow obstruction. Br J Urol 57:657–659

Raz S, Ziegler M, Caine M (1973) Pharmacologic receptors in the prostate. Br J Urol 45:663

Ronchi F, Margonato A, Ceccardi R et al. (1982) Symptomatic treatment of benign prostatic obstruction with nicergoline: a placebo-controlled clinical study and urodynamic evaluation. Urol Res 10:131–134

Rudd P (1986) Cumulative experience with terazosin administered in combination with diuretics. Am J Med 80 [Suppl 5B]: 49–54

Scott MA, Abrams P (1989) Indoramin in the treatment of prostatic bladder outflow obstruction. Neurol Urodyn 8:217

Shapiro E, Lepor H (1987) Alpha adrenergic receptors in canine lower genitourinary tissues: insight into development and function. J Urol 138:979–984

Shapiro E, Becich MJ, Lepor H (1992) The relative proportion of stromal and epithelial hyperplasia is related to the development of clinical BPH J Urol (in press)

Flutamide and Aromatase Inhibitors in Benign Prostatic Hypertrophy

N.N.Stone

Introduction

Benign prostatic hypertrophy (BPH) is an age related phenomenon in which hormonal regulation has a significant role. While the exact nature of the influence of either androgens or estrogens remains unresolved, there is ample evidence to support their pharmacologic manipulation in the treatment of BPH. Hormonal regulation of BPH can be initiated by one of several approaches:

1. Decreasing of available dihydrotestosterone (DHT) by blocking the conversion of testosterone (T) to DHT by a 5α-reductase inhibitor or by castration
2. Preventing binding of either T or DHT to the receptor by an antiandrogen
3. Preventing the action of estrogens by an antiestrogen or by decreasing available estrogen by blocking its production with an aromatase inhibitor

This chapter will discuss the use of flutamide, an antiandrogen, and aromatase inhibitors in BPH.

Flutamide

Flutamide (α-α-α-trifluoro-2-methyl-4′-nitro-m-propionotoluidide) is a nonsteroidal antiandrogen which is metabolized into a hydroxylated derivative that competitively competes with either T or DHT for cytosol androgen receptor sites (Liao et al. 1974, Figs. 1–2). With oral dosing, flutamide is rapidly absorbed and excreted mainly through the kidneys (Katchen and Buxbaum 1975). It is highly protein bound and has a half-life of about 8 h.

Studies of androgen deprivation with flutamide in the rat and canine support its use in treating both BPH and prostate cancer (Neri et al. 1972). When given at a dose range of 5–50 mg/kg in dogs for 6 weeks, a significant decrease in prostate volume and in epithelial cell height was noted (Neri and Monahan 1972). Further reduction in prostate volume and epithelial cell height occurred for up to 1 year, suggesting the lengthy process required to achieve prostate gland involution. The favorable results from the animal studies eventually led to designing human clinical trials.

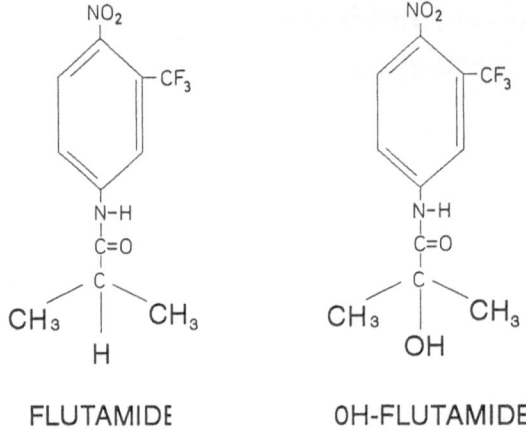

Fig. 1. Structure of flutamide and the active metabolic compound hydroxyflutamide

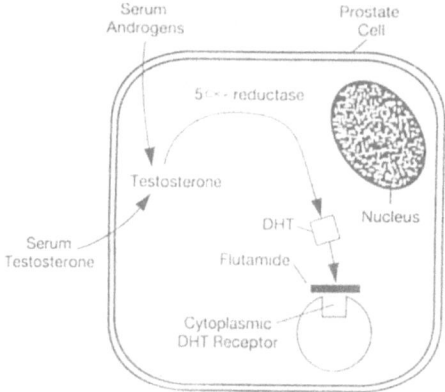

Fig. 2. Method of action of antiandrogen flutamide. (From Stone 1989)

The minimal toxicity experienced with flutamide in these animal studies implied that it might be a safe and acceptable compound in men. While it is known that castration will result in impotence and decreased libido, the animal studies using flutamide as the means of achieving androgen deprivation showed no such side effects (Neri and Peets 1975). Thus, flutamide's antiandrogen activity could be utilized without sacrificing potency – clearly a major advantage in treating patients with BPH.

Clinical studies on the use of flutamide for prostatic diseases have been limited. More data are available on flutamide monotherapy for prostate cancer than for BPH and thus a brief review on the use of flutamide in patients with prostate cancer is worthwhile.

Flutamide monotherapy studies were attempted in patients with newly diagnosed stage D2 prostate cancer with the hope of offering androgen deprivation without the side effects of impotence. Sogani studied 80 men with advanced prostate cancer and found a 70% response rate and preservation of potency in most of the patients (Sogani et al. 1984). However, significant side effects including gynecomastia did occur. The greatest concern with this method of androgen ablation was generated in a small study of 11 patients in whom serum T levels were noted to rise with continued administration of flutamide. The increased T could potentially lead to tumor escape, and thus further monotherapy with flutamide for prostate cancer was eventually limited (Hellman et al. 1977).

The rising T is caused by the binding of flutamide to the androgen receptor in the gonadotroph cells. This leads to an increase in lutenizing hormone (LH) levels which occurs in the face of high T concentrations (Neri et al. 1972; Poyet and Labrie 1985). The higher LH levels result from both an increase in LH synthesis and release (Knuth et al. 1984; Sardanons et al. 1989). Because flutamide is a competitive inhibitor, the rising T level could potentially compromise the androgen blockade and theoretically permit disease progression. However, long-term use of flutamide monotherapy in patients with prostate cancer does not appear to result in chronically elevated serum T levels (Lund and Rasmussen 1988). Nevertheless, because of these initial concerns, flutamide monotherapy for prostate cancer was not actively pursued in the United States.

The concept of using flutamide for patients with BPH was first introduced by Caine. In a double-blind trial 30 patients were given 300 mg of flutamide or placebo for 12 weeks (Caine et al. 1975). Significant improvements were noted in the flutamide group in maximum and average uroflow rates. No benefit was found with changes in prostate gland size, but, as the size of the prostate gland was assessed by digital rectal exam and not ultrasound, only large changes would be expected to have been detected. Treated patients also noted symptom improvements. However, while the symptom improvements were statistically significant at 8 weeks, by the end of the study they were not different from placebo.

While Caine's study was pivotal in demonstrating the use of antiandrogen therapy for BPH, it resulted in raising more questions than it answered. Unfortunately, a phase III trial was chosen when neither the correct dose nor the appropriate duration of administration were known. Extrapolation from the canine data suggests that too low a dose (<5 mg/kg) for too short a period (<24 weeks) was used in Caine's study. More recent studies with androgen deprivation using lutenizing hormone releasing hormone against (LHRHa) compounds confirm that a minimum of 4–6 months is needed to achieve maximum prostate gland size reduction (Gabrilove et al. 1987; Peters and Walsh 1987). The most appropriate dose of flutamide for BPH is still not known because no dose ranging studies with flutamide have been reported.

Despite these shortcomings, Caine was able to show the potential to use flutamide in patients with BPH. Toxicity was low and gynecomastia or mastalgia occured in seven of 15 patients. No patients reported loss of potency.

Because of the increased interest in medical therapy for BPH, an industry-sponsored, randomized, controlled study of flutamide was initiated in the United States. Patients were randomized to either 750 mg of flutamide/day (250mg t.i.d.)

or placebo. A total of 84 patients were enrolled (42 placebo, 42 flutamide) and response were analyzed for changes in prostate volume, uroflow rates, and symptom scores (Stone 1989).

Significant improvements were noted in all parameters in the treated group. Prostate volume decreased a median of 18% by 3 months and 41% by 6 months. Uroflow increased by 35% in the treated group, while no improvement was noted in the patients on placebo. Both groups of patients had a 50% improvement in overall symptom scores (Figs. 3, 4).

As might be expected, there was a significantly higher proportion of adverse reactions reported in the flutamide group. For the most part, these side effects were mild and did not cause patients to drop out of the study. While 53% of the patients noted some breast pain or gynecomastia, only one patient (3%) reported this as being more than mild. Four patients noted diarrhea (11%) and again only one (3%) stated that this was more than mild. No patients complained of impotence or decreased libido as a result of taking flutamide.

A more recent report analyzed the effect of flutamide on prostate volume, prostate-specific antigen (PSA), and T in men with BPH (Stone and Clejan 1991). In 11 patients who received flutamide for 6 months, prostate volume decreased

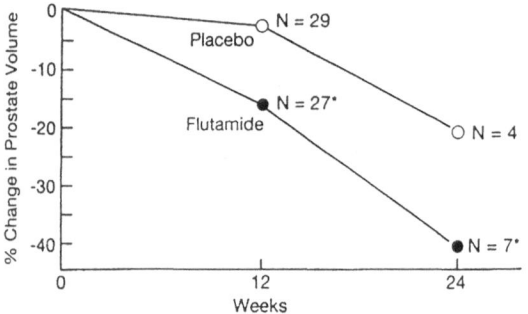

Fig. 3. Median percent change in prostate volume in patients on flutamide or placebo ($^*p < 0.01$). (From Stone 1989)

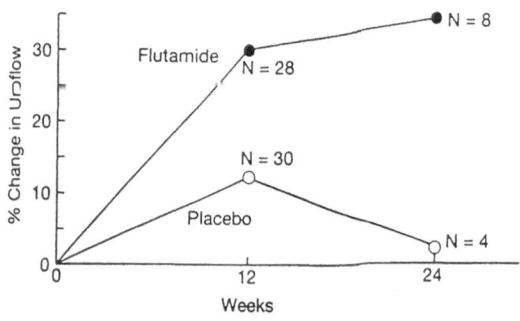

Fig. 4. Median percent change in uroflow. (From Stone 1989)

from a mean of 101 cm³ to 66 cm³ (mean decrease 35%) and serum PSA decreased
from 10.7 ng/ml to 3.8 ng/ml (mean decrease 65%). These changes occured despite
an increase in serum T from a mean of 336 ng/dl to 518 ng/dl (mean increase
58.3%) (Fig. 5). Thus, despite an increase in T, flutamide was able to continue to
maintain a state of androgen deprivation. Side effects were similar in this study
with 36% complaining of mild gynecomastia and one patient reporting a decrease
in potency.

There is compelling evidence that suggests that flutamide may eventually be an
important agent in treating BPH. Other newer antiandrogens such as casodex or
zanoterone are currently under clinical study and may further add to the number
of agents to treat BPH. These compounds are reported to have greater potency,
improved tolerance, longer half-life, and to be less likely to raise LH levels when
compared to flutamide (Kennealey and Furr 1991). Whether these or other newer

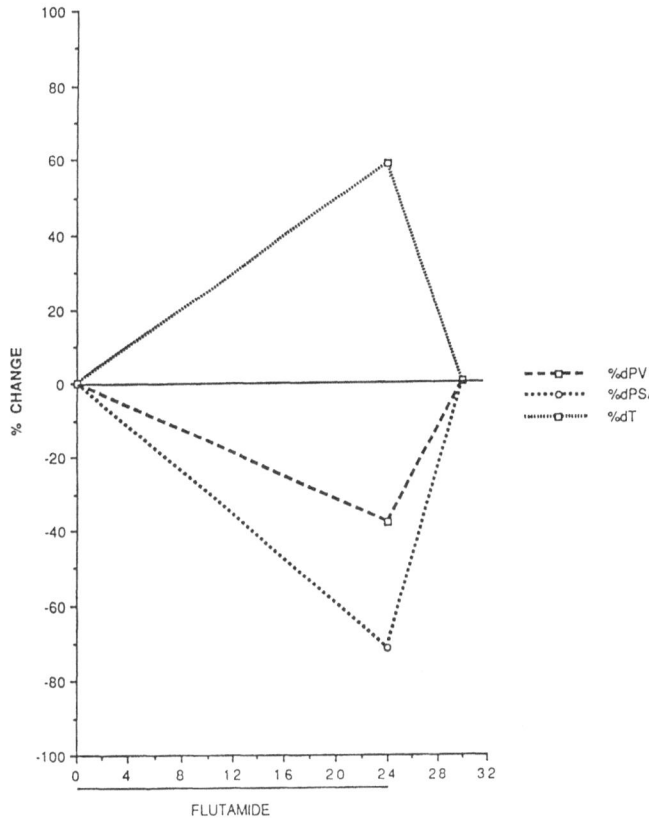

Fig. 5. Mean percent change in prostate volume (*%dPV*), prostate-specific antigen (*%dPSA*), and testosterone (*%dT*) in patients with BPH on flutamide for 24 weeks and off for 6 weeks. (From Stone and
Clejan 1991)

agents will be as effective as flutamide in treating BPH and have less toxicity still needs to be determined by clinical trials.

Aromatase Inhibitors

Estrogen formation results from the aromatization of androgens in a P450-dependent enzyme system at several sites (Fig. 6).

The conversion of androstenedione to estrone involves three hydroxylations, at C-19$_1$, C-19$_2$, and C-2$_\beta$. The collapse of the resultant 2$_\beta$-hydroxy-19-oxoandrostenedione yields the aromatic A-ring of estrone and thus the process is referred to as aromatization (Fishman 1982; Fishman and Goto 1981).

In the male, estrogen biosynthesis has been demonstrated in the testis, skin fibroblasts, adipose and muscle tissue, hair follicles, liver, brain, and prostate (Schweikert 1979; Schweikert et al. 1975; Folkerd and James 1983; Longcope et al. 1978; Fishman and Goto 1981; Stone et al. 1986, 1987). Estrogen production in men ranges from 100–400 pmole/day.

The exact role that estrogens may have in the pathogenesis and maintenance of BPH is not fully known. However, the importance of estrogens as a cofactor in BPH genesis is well characterized in experimental models. Induction of BPH in castrate

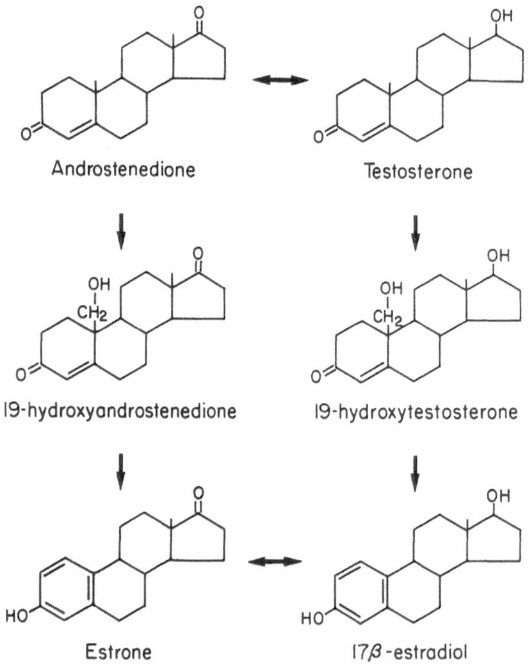

Androstenedione	Testosterone
19-hydroxyandrostenedione	19-hydroxytestosterone
Estrone	17β-estradiol

Fig. 6. Formation of estrone and estradiol from androgen precursors

dogs with DHT and estradiol has been extensively studied and has demonstrated great synergism (DeKlerk et al. 1979; Walsh and Wilson 1976; Habenicht and El Etreby 1987; Habenicht et al. 1986a,b).

Other evidence exists that suggests estrogens may be involved in more than a supportive role in BPH. The presence of high estrogen levels in stromal nuclei in patients with BPH (Kozak et al. 1982; Krieg et al. 1987), the positive mitogenic effect of estrogens on fibroblasts (Mawhinney and Neubauer 1979), the influence of estrogens on androgen receptor content regulation (Bouton et al. 1981; Trachtenberg et al. 1980), and the effect of the antiestrogen tamoxifen on stromal protein synthesis in the human prostate (Liu et al. 1984) all lend evidence to the possibility that manipulation of the native estrogen environment might potentially affect BPH status.

The issue of whether the prostate gland itself may be involved in estrogen synthesis and itself contribute to BPH genesis by autocrine regulation is controversial. Estrogen biosynthesis in the prostate was first identified by Schweikert when estrogen formation was demonstrated in cultured prostate stromal fibroblasts (Schweikert 1979). Activity was again demonstrated by Stone in an invitro assay of BPH tissue vs non-BPH tissue (Fig. 7, Stone et al. 1986, 1987).

Table 1 shows the results of several different investigations of prostate aromatization. The results vary from no formation to a high of 223 fmol/mg protein/h. Thus, the issue of prostate gland auto-regulation of BPH by in situ estrogen formation is yet to be resolved.

Estrogen deprivation therapy was probably first practiced at the turn of the century when orchiectomy was performed for BPH (Cabot 1896; White 1895).

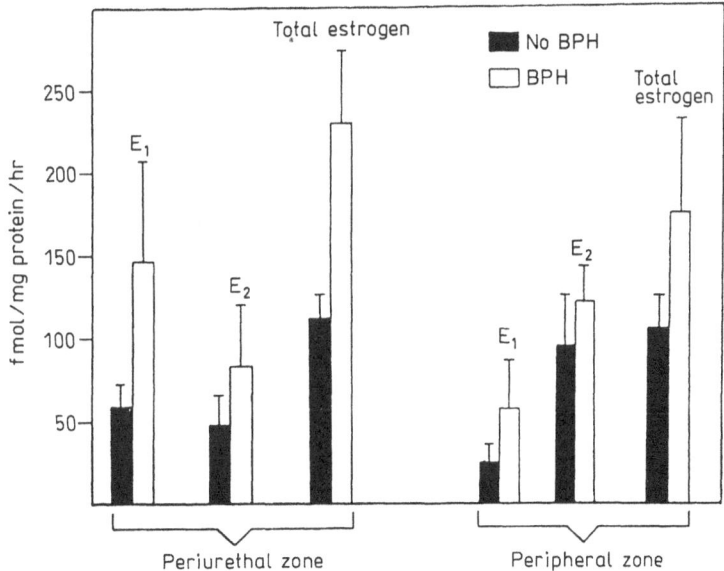

Fig. 7. Estrogen formation in human prostatic tissue with and without BPH. (From Stone et al. 1986)

Table 1. Estrogen production in the prostate

Reference	Tissue source	Rate of estrogen production
Schweikert and Tunn (1987)	Prostate fibroblasts	30–116 fmol/mg protein/h
Stone (1989)	BPH homogenates	223 fmol/mg protein/h
Kabugari et al. (1987)	BPH homogenates	23.6 fmol/250 mg prostate/h
Smith et al. (1982)	BPH homogenates	None
Broide et al. (1989)	BPH homogenates	None
Bartsch et al. (1987)	BPH homogenates	$< 7 \times 10^{-17}$ mol/mg protein/min

Although not realized at the time, castration not only reduced serum androgen levels, but also greatly lowered estrogen levels. This relationship was demonstrated in the contemporary LHRHa studies in which serum hormones levels were determined in men with BPH who were treated with these agents (Gabrilove et al. 1987). Thus the beneficial effect of castration on BPH may be due to both estrogen and androgen deprivation.

Studies on the use of aromatase inhibitors to manipulate BPH have yielded controversial results. While there is little controversy on the enhancing effect estrogens have on canine BPH, the reversibility of existing BPH with such agents has not been extensively studied.

The potential for using such compounds can be inferred from canine studies (Fig. 8). The antiestrogen effects of the aromatase inhibitors 4-hydroxy-4-androstene-3,-17-dione (4-OH-AD) and 1-methyl-1,-4-androstadiene-3, 17-dione (atamestane) have been studied in the dog with BPH and support the potential use of these agents in humans (Habenicht et al. 1986 a, b).

Castrated beagles were treated with androstenedione alone or in combination with atamestane (Habenicht and El Etreby 1987). There was a significant increase

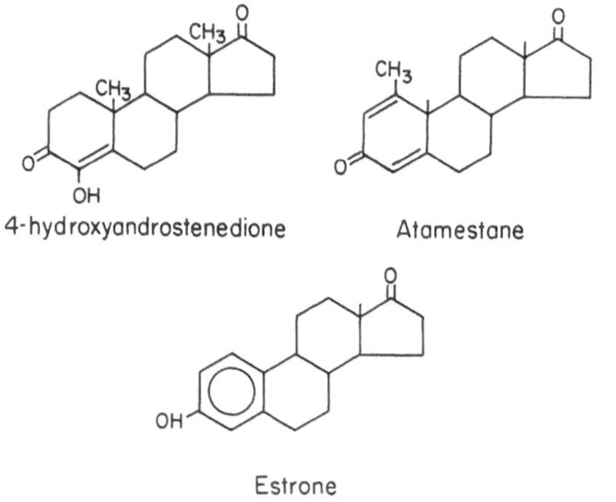

4-hydroxyandrostenedione   Atamestane

Estrone

Fig. 8. Structure of two aromatase inhibitors 4-hydroxy-androstenedione (4OH-AD) and atamestane compared to estrone

in prostate weight in the castrated animals treated with androstenedione which was antagonized by atamestane. The prostate of animals treated with the aromatase inhibitor were also characterized by inhibition of the stroma, including smooth muscle.

In contrast to the above studies which were performed in castrate dogs, in which the induction of BPH was inhibited by combining an aromatizable androgen (androstenedione) with an aromatase inhibitor, studies with the use of an aromatase inhibitor in intact beagles with existing BPH have not produced such positive results. Male animals were administered an orally active nonsteroidal aromatase inhibitor, 4-(5,6,7,8-tetrahydro-imidazo [1,5α] pyridin-5-yl) benzonitrile hydrochloride (CGS 16949A, Ciba-Geigy Corp, Summit, NJ), with the intent of lowering estrogen levels and reversing existing BPH. This study found that after 25 weeks of treatment no significant changes occurred in prostatic weight or total DNA content. While a tenfold rise in serum T was found, no significant changes were noted in prostatic tissue concentrations of T, DHT, or 5α-androstan-3α, 17β-diol. The authors concluded that aromatase inhibitors could not be effectively utilized to treat existing BPH (Juniewicz et al. 1988; Oesterling et al. 1988).

Clinical studies with aromatase inhibitors in men with BPH have been limited. Prostate volume was found to decrease an average of 26% in 13 patients in urinary retention treated with testolactone (100 mg b.i.d. for 6 months). These 13 patients were in urinary retention and seven resolved the retention while on the testolactone (Schweikert and Tunn 1987).

Clinical data is rapidly becoming available on the aromatase inhibitor atamestane. Atamestane is a competitive aromatase inhibitor with no affinity to steroid receptors (El Etreby et al. 1991).

Human pharmacodynamic studies suggest few side effects and high effectiveness in lowering estrogen concentrations (El Etreby et al. 1991). Seven days of treatment with 5–10 mg/kg atamestane in patients with BPH resulted in lowering serum estrogen levels between 22% and 76%. While there was a significant decrease in intraprostatic estrone levels with atamestane, prostatic estradiol levels were unchanged. In addition a slight rise in serum T and DHT was found after 7 days administration. Whether this will compromise the effectiveness of this compound in treating BPH is currently being determined in phase II clinical trials.

BPH should not be regarded as one disease. It is clear from a histologic stand point that elements more responsive to androgen deprivation (glandular hyperplasia) and elements potentially more responsive to estrogen deprivation (stromal hyperplasia) coexist within the prostate. It may be that identification of individual histological patterns (Newman et al. 1991) could improve treatment choices or that combination therapy (antiandrogen/5α-reductase inhibitor plus aromatase inhibitor) would favour improved clinical results. Once the clinical efficacy and safety of the individual compounds have been demonstrated, the potential to use combination therapy can then be investigated.

References

Bartsch W, Klein H, Sturenburg H-J, Voigt K-D (1987) Metabolism of androgens in human benign prostatic hyperplasia: aromatase and its inhibition. J Steroid Biochem 27:557–564

Bouton MM, Porin C, Grandadan JA (1981) Estrogen regulation of rat prostate androgen receptor. J Steroid Biochem 15:403–408

Brodie AMH, Son C, King DA, Meyer KM, Inkster SE (1989) Lack of evidence of aromatase in human prostatic tissues: effects of 4-hydroxy androstenedione and other inhibitors of androgen metabolism. Cancer Res. 49:6551–6555

Cabot AT (1896) The question of castration for enlarged prostate. Ann Surg 24:265–301

Caine M, Perlberg S, Gordon R (1975) The Treatment of Benign Prostatic Hypertrophy with Flutamide (SCH 13521): A Placebo-Controlled Study. J Urol 114:564–568

DeKlerk DP, Coffey DS, Ewing LL, McDermott IR, Reiner WG, Robinson CH, Scott WW, Strandberg JD, Talaloy P, Walsh PC, Wheaton LG, Zirkin BR (1979) Comparison of spontaneous and experimentally induced canine prostatic hyperplasia. J Clin Invest 168:842–849

El Etreby MF, Nishino Y, Habenicht UF, Henderson D (1991) Atamestane, a new aromatase inhibitor for the management of benign prostate hyperplasia. J Androl 12:403–414

Fishman J (1982) Biochemical mechanisms of aromatization. Cancer Res 42:3277s–3279s

Fishman J, Goto J (1981) Mechanism of estrogen biosynthesis. J Biological Chem 256:4466–4471

Folkerd EJ, James VHT (1983) Aromatization of steroids in peripheral tissues. J Steroid Biochem 49:687–690

Gabrilove JL, Levine AC, Kirschenbaum A, Droller MJ (1987) Effect of a GNRH analogue (leuprolide) on benign prostate hypertrophy. J Clin Endocrinol Metab 64:1331–1333

Geller J, Albert J, Nachtscheim DA, Loza D, Geller S (1981) The effects of flutamide on total DHT and nuclear DHT levels in the human prostate. Prostate 2:309–314

Habenicht UF, El Etreby MF (1987) Synergic inhibitory effects of the aromatase inhibitor 1-methyl-antrosta-1, 4-dione-3, 17 dione and the androstenedione-induced hyperplastic effects in the prostates of castrate dogs. Prostate 11:133–143

Habenicht UF, Schwartz K, Schweikert HU, Neumann F, El Etreby MF (1986a) Development of a model for the induction of estrogen related to prostatic hyperplasia in the dog and its response to the aromatase inhibitor 4-hydroxy-4-androstene-3, 17-dione: preliminary results. Prostate 8: 181–194

Habenicht UF, El Etreby MF, Tunn UW, Schweikert HU, Neumann F (1986b) Animal models for investigating the role of oestrogens in the pathogenesis of benign prostatic hyperplasia. In: Di Silverio I, Neumann F, Tannenbaum M (eds) Ipertrofia Prostatica Benigna. Elsevier, Amsterdam, pp 81–77

Hellman L, Bradalow HL, Freed S, Levin J, Rosenfeld RS, Whitmore WF, Zumoff B (1977) The Effect of Flutamide on Testosterone Metabolism and the Plasma Levels of Androgens and gonadotropins. J Clin Endocrin Metab 45:1224–1229

Juniewicz PE, Oesterling JE, Walters JR, Steele RE, Niswender GD, Coffey DS, Ewing LL (1988) Aromatase inhibitor in the dog. I Effect on Serum LH, Serum Testosterone Concentrations, Testicular Secretions and Spermatogenesis. J Urol 139:827–831

Kaburagi Y, Marino MB, Kirdanc RY, Greco JP, Karr JP, Sandberg, AA (1987) The possibility of aromatization of androgen in human prostate. J Steroid Biochem 26:739–742

Karr JP, Kaburagi Y, Mann CF, Sandberg AA (1987) The potential significance of aromatase in the etiology and treatment of prostatic disease. Steroids 50:4–5

Katchen B, Buxbaum S (1975) Disposition of a New, Nonsteroid, Antiandrogen, a a-a-Trifluoro 2 methyl-4'-nitro-m-propionotoluide (Flutamide), in Men Following a Single Oral 200mg Dose. J Clin Endocrinol Metab 41:373–379

Kennealey GT, Furr BJA (1991) Use of the nonsteroidal anti-androgen casodex in advanced prostate cancer. Urol Clin North Am 18: 99–110

Knuth UA, Hano R, Nieschlag E (1984) Effect of flutamide or cyproterone acetate on pituitary and testicular hormones in normal men. J Clin Endocrinol Metab 59:963–969

Kozak I, Bartsch W, Krieg M, Voigt KD (1982) Nuclei of stroma: Site of highest estrogen concentration in human benign prostatic hyperplasia. The Prostate 3:433–438

Krieg M, Bartsch W, Thompson M, Voigt KD (1983) Androgens and estrogens: Their interaction with stroma and epithelium of human benign prostatic hyperplasia and normal prostate. J Steroid Biochem 19:155–161

Liao S, Howell DK, Chung T (1974) Action of a nonsteroidal antiandrogen, flutamide, on the receptor binding and nuclear retention of 5 a-dihydrotestosterone in rat ventral prostate. Endocrinology 94:1205–1209

Liu J, Albert JD, Geller J, Faber LE (1984) Effect of Tamoxifen on stromal protein synthesis in human prostate. J Clin Endocrinol Metab 59:710–713

Longcope C, Pratt JH, Scheider SH, Fineberg SE (1978) Aromatization of androgens by muscle and adipose tissue in vivo. J Clin Endocrinol Metab 46:146–152

Lund F, Rasmussen F (1988) Flutamide versus stilbesterol in the management of advanced prostate cancer. Br J Urol 61:140–142

Mawhinney MG, Neubauer BL (1979) Actions of estrogen in the male. Invest Urol 16:409–420

Neri RO, Monahan M (1972) Effects of a novel nonsteroidal antiandrogen on canine prostatic hyperplasia. Invest Urol 10:123–130

Neri RO, Peets EA (1975) Biological aspects of antiandrogens. J Steriod Biochem 6:815–819

Neri RO, Florence K, Koziol P, Cleave S J (1972) Abiological Profile of a nonsteroidal Antiandrogen, Sch 13321 (4'-nitro-3'-trifluorethylisobatyranilide). Endocrinology 91:427–437

Newman LH, Stone, NN Waxman JS, Lau TS, Chen G (1991) Determination of prostate glandular content by prostate volume and prostate specific antigen. J Urol 145:216a

Oesterling JE, Juniewicz PE, Walters JR, Strandberg JD, Steele RE, Ewing LL, Coffey DS (1988) Aromatase inhibitor in the dog. II. Effect on serum LH, serum testosterone concentrations, testicular secretions and spermatogenesis. J Urol 139:832–839

Peters CA, Walsh PC (1987) The effect of naferlin acetate, a luteinizing hormone-releasing hormone agonist, on benign prostate hyperplasia. N Engl J Med 317:599–604

Poyet P, Labrie F (1985) Comparison of the antiandrogenic/androgenic activities of flutamide, cyproterone acetate and megestrol acetate. Mol Cell Endocrinol 42:283–288

Sardanons ML, Heras Ma delas, Calandra RS, Solano AR, Podesta EJ (1989) Effect of the antiandrogen flutamide o pituitary LH content and release. Neuroendocrinology 50:211–216

Schweikert HU (1979) Conversion of androstenedione to estrone in human fibroblasts cultured from prostate, genitals and non-genital skin. Hormone Metab Res 11:635–640

Schweikert HU, Milewich L, Wilson, JD (1975) Aromatization of androstenedione by isolated human hairs. J Clin Endocrinol Metab 40:413–417

Schweikert HU, Tunn UW (1987) Effects of the aromatase inhibitor testolactone on human benign prostatic hyperplasia. Steroids 50:1–3

Sogani PC, Vagaiwala MR, Whitmore WF (1984) Experience with flutamide in patients with advanced prostate cancer without prior endocrine therapy. Cancer 54:744–750

Smith T, Chisholm GD, Habib FK (1982) Failure of human benign prostatic hyperplasia to aromatase testosterone. J Steroid Biochem 17:119–120

Stone NN (1989) Flutamide in treatment of benign prostate hypertrophy. Urology [Suppl] 34:64–68

Stone NN, Clejan SJ (1991) Response of prostate volume, prostate-specific antigen, and testosterone to flutamide in men with benign prostate hyperplasia. J Androl 12:376–380

Stone NN, Fair W, Fishman J (1986) Estrogen formation in human prostatic tissue from patients with and without benign prostatic hyperplasia. Prostate 9:34

Stone NN, Laudone V, Fair W, Fishman J (1987) Aromatization of androstenedione by benign prostatic hyperplasia, prostate cancer and expressed prostatic secretions. Urol Res 15:165–167

Trachtenberg J, Hicks LL, Walsh PC (1980) Androgen and estrogen-receptor content in spontaneous and experimentally induced canine prostatic hyperplasia. J Clin Invest 65:1051–1059

Walsh PC, Wilson JD (1976) The induction of prostatic hyperthrophy in the dog with androstanediol. J Clin Invest 57:1093–1097

White JW (1895) The result of double castration in hypertrophy of the prostate. Ann Surg 22:1–59

Finasteride: A 5α-Reductase Inhibitor

E.Stoner, E.Round, and P.Grino

Introduction

In selected male reproductive organs, such as the prostate, testosterone (T) is converted to the more potent androgen dihydrotestosterone (DHT) by the enzyme 5α-reductase (5α-R). DHT is currently regarded as the most important factor in the pathogenesis of benign prostatic hyperplasia (BPH). This is based on experimental data showing that DHT is by far the most abundant androgenic hormone within prostatic cell nuclei (Bruchovsky and Wilson 1968) and the observation that men with the genetic syndrome of 5α-R deficiency (male pseudohermaphrodites, MPHs) have atrophic prostate glands throughout their lives (Imperato-McGinley et al. 1974; Walsh et al. 1974).

Imperato-McGinley recently summarized some of the striking clinical findings in MPHs with 5α-R deficiency (1991). Affected prepubertal subjects have separate vaginal and urethral openings within a urogenital sinus, and a clitoris-like phallus. Because the developmental defect is limited to the external genitalia, Imperato-McGinley proposes that its differentiation is mediated by DHT. In contrast, differentiation of the Wolffian ducts, which appears to be mediated by T, proceeds normally in male fetuses with 5α-R deficiency, as demonstrated by the presence of epididymides, vasa deferentia, and seminal vesicles. Scrotal development, penile enlargement, muscle mass, and libido develop normally at puberty indicating that these effects are primarily mediated by T.

However, throughout adult life certain tissues, such as the prostate gland and skin structures, which should normally contain high levels of 5α-R, remain affected by the genetic deficiency; the prostate remains small, facial and body hair remain scanty, and severe acne or temporal recession of the hairline do not occur. Thus it appears that 5α-R is responsible for the normal development of the external male genitalia in utero, the development of secondary sexual characteristics at puberty, and the maintenance of these characteristic and growth of the prostate gland in adulthood.

These observations provided a model that would predict the biologic effects of chronic 5α-R inhibition in adult men, suggesting that specific inhibition of this enzyme might decrease DHT formation within the prostate and result in involution of hyperplastic tissue in patients with BPH.

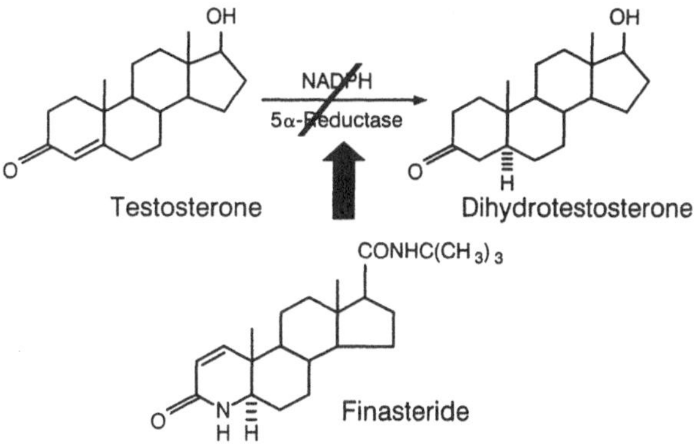

Fig. 1. Mechanism of action for finasteride, reprinted from J. Steroid Biochem. Molec. Biol. (1990), 37: 375–378. Pergamon Press Ltd.

Research scientists at Merck Research Laboratories hypothesized that a compound could be formulated that would selectively inhibit the enzyme 5α-R without affecting the binding of T or DHT to the androgen receptor. Through such selectivity, it would be possible to effectively treat BPH without the feminizing side effects, such as gynecomastia, impotence, and loss of libido seen with androgen receptor antagonists.

Finasteride (MK-906, PROSCAR), a specific inhibitor of 5α-R, blocks the conversion of T to DHT vitro and in in vivo and is the first such compound to be clinically evaluated in men with BPH (Fig. 1).

Preclinical Studies

Animal studies have demonstrated that finasteride is devoid of androgenic, antiandrogenic, or other steroid hormone-related properties (Stoner 1990). When male rats were treated with finasteride from birth to puberty, George et al. (1989) observed that by 7 weeks of age, blood T levels increased more than sevenfold while the circulating DHT level declined. In these rats, tissue weights of prostate, penis, seminal vesicles, and epididymides were 30%–50% lower than those of the controls. The investigators emphasized that treatment with finasteride did not affect testicular histology or sperm production despite significant reductions in intratesticular DHT and significant increases in intratesticular T. They concluded that DHT is not critical for normal spermatogenesis or for the development of preputial glands or androgen-dependent perineal muscles in rats.

Brooks et al. (1982, 1986) also demonstrated that mature beagles had significant reductions in prostate size when treated with finasteride.

Clinical Studies: Healthy Volunteers

The biochemical activity, safety, tolerability, and clinical efficacy of finasteride have been studied in humans since March 1986. In Phase I clinical studies of 54 healthy volunteers, Vermeulen et al. (1989) demonstrated that a single oral dose of 0.5 mg decreased plasma DHT levels by 65% after 24 h, thus confirming the biochemical efficacy and potency of finasteride.

In addition, a single dose of 10 mg of finasteride was shown to suppress androstanediol glucuronide and androsterone glucuronide formation (Rittmaster et al. 1989), which suggests that the formation of both conjugated and unconjugated 5α-reduced androgens is suppressed by finasteride in hepatic and extrasplanchnic tissues.

A double-blind placebo-controlled trial comparing the efficacy of high- (25–100 mg) and low-dose (0.04–1.0 mg) finasteride administered in daily oral doses for 11 and 14 days, respectively, showed a significant reduction in DHT at all doses, including the lowest dose of 0.04 mg (Gormley et al. 1989). Treatment did not affect follicle-stimulating hormone (FSH), cortisol, estradiol, or serum lipids, such as total cholesterol, LDL, HDL, and triglycerides (Table 1).

These studies clearly established that finasteride caused a significant decrease in circulating DHT in normal volunteers which was reversed when treatment was withdrawn.

Table 1. Metabolic Effects of Finasteride

Clinically significant reduction in:
  Serum and intraprostatic DHT
  Serum and intraprostatic PSA

Significant increase in:
  Intraprostatic testosterone

No clinically significant change in serum:
  Testosterone
  LH or FSH
  Cortisol
  Prolactin
  Estradiol
  Thyroid function
  Lipid profile
  Glucose tolerance
  Routine biochemistry or hematology

DHT, dihydrotestosterone; PSA, prostate-specific antigen.

Phase II Clinical Studies: Patients

Hormonal Effects

In a double-blind placebo-controlled trial of 69 men with BPH, finasteride (1, 5, 10, 50, or 100 mg) was administered for 7 days prior to transurethral resection of the prostate (McConnell et al. 1992). The investigators determined that a 1×5 mg dose decreased intraprostatic DHT by approximately 87%, from 10.3 ± 0.6 nmol/kg ($\pm$ SE) to 1.4 ± 0.3 nmol/kg, while intraprostatic T increased by approximately sixfold (from 0.7 ± 0.1 nmol/kg to 4.4 ± 0.8 nmol/kg).

Furthermore, a marked decrease in intraprostatic levels of prostate-specific antigen (PSA) has been found in BPH patients receiving finasteride (50 and 100 mg) for 1 week before surgery (Geller and Franson 1989). A significant correlation ($y \pm 0.83$) between prostatic PSA content and prostate epithelial cell DHT levels was also observed in this study.

Clinical studies in BPH patients treated for 6 months confirmed a marked decrease in circulating DHT; in fact, a 5 mg dose of finasteride achieved 80% suppression of circulating DHT, similar to that observed following castration (Stoner 1990). Other circulating hormones, such as luteinizing hormone (LH), cortisol, prolactin, and estradiol, remained unchanged.

In a comparison of the 5α-steroid metabolite profile between men with 5α-R deficiency and normal subjects treated with finasteride, Imperato-McGinley (1991) showed that finasteride causes an alteration in steroid metabolism similar to the genetic deficiency. Finasteride effectively blocks the 5α-reduction of steroids other than T and a more profound lowering of serum DHT was observed than that seen in the genetic syndrome.

Effects on Prostate Volume and Urinary Flow Rate

In a 6 month placebo-controlled study of patients with BPH, prostate volume decreased in the finasteride group by a mean of 18% in 3 months and 27% in 6 months (Stoner et al. 1992). Prostate shrinkage in the placebo group was less than 7%. At the end of the study, the mean increase in urinary flow rate was about 3.8 ml/s compared with no increase in the placebo group. These data suggested that, although early improvement has been seen, a treatment period of at least 6 months may be required to achieve a maximum therapeutic response.

In order to confirm whether these effects would be maintained with chronic therapy, a 1 year extension study of 67 patients (mean age: 66 years) with BPH was undertaken (Finasteride Study Group 1991). All patients had documented prostatic enlargement (baseline prostate volume: 80.8 cm^3) and symptoms of lower urinary tract obstruction. After receiving finasteride 10 mg once daily for 6 months the mean prostate volume was 67.6 cm^3 and was further reduced to 62.3 cm^3 after 12 months.

In addition, patients whose baseline maximum urinary flow rates were less than 15 ml/s experienced a mean increase in maximum urinary flow rate of 4 ml/s by month 12; about 70% of these patients had a minimum of 3 ml/s improvement in maximum urinary flow rate. No drug-related adverse effects were reported throughout the trial period.

A placebo-controlled study of finasteride (PROSCAR Study Group 1991) was conducted in a total of 104 patients, in which the treated group received single daily doses ranging from 0.2 to 40 mg for 6 months. Of the original group of patients, 88 entered a 12 month open extension, receiving 5 mg daily. Prostate volume, measured by magnetic resonance imaging (MRI), was reduced in the finasteride group by 26% during the first 6 months of the study, compared with a 5% reduction in the placebo group. This reduction was maintained throughout the 18 month study period.

In treated patients with baseline maximum urinary flow rates less than 15 ml/s, a 3.5 ml/s increase in maximum urinary flow rate was obtained, which was maintained throughout the extension period. In contrast, no increase in maximum urinary flow rate occurred in the placebo-treated patients. A beneficial effect on symptoms was seen in the finasteride group and maintained throughout the course of the trial.

Overview of Phase III Trials

To date, the most important data on the use of finasteride in the treatment of BPH are derived from two, large-scale, multicenter, double-blind, placebo-controlled, Phase III trials, known as the North American (895 patients) and International (750 patients) studies conducted by the Finasteride Study Group (1992a,b).

Two differences in the study design existed between the trials: In the North American study, prostate volume was measured by MRI, and there were no entry requirements for minimum prostate volume. In the International study, transrectal ultrasonography (TRUS) was used to determine prostate volume and only patients with prostates larger than 30 g were entered. Both studies required patients to have a baseline maximum urinary flow rate of less than 15 ml/s for entry. Finasteride-treated patients were given either 1 or 5 mg once daily for 12 months.

Hormonal Effects

As was expected, there was a dramatic and sustained decrease in plasma DHT. LH and T levels increased slightly but did not exceed the normal range. A 40%–50% median reduction was observed in plasma PSA, a marker of prostatic epithelial tissue cell activity.

Effects on Prostate Volume and Urinary Flow Rate

Both doses of finasteride reduced prostate volume by about 20% compared with placebo. However, placebo-treated patients had an initial increase in maximum urinary flow rate, which then plateaued over the next 11 months. Finasteride-treated patients showed a progressive trend toward urinary flow improvement and by month 12 achieved a mean increase in maximum urinary flow rate of 1.5 ml/s. Residual urine volume decreased in all treatment groups from baseline, but there were no significant differences among them at the end of the study.

Effects on Symptoms

A striking placebo effect was observed on symptoms as assessed by a questionnaire that included both obstructive and irritative symptoms. During the first few months of the study placebo-treated patients reported improvements in their symptoms, after this the improvement halted and significant differences in symptom score were observed between patients treated with 5 mg finasteride, compared with placebo. After 9 months, the finasteride-treated group showed a further improvement in symptoms, resulting in statistically significant differences from placebo by the end of the study ($p < .01$). When compared with a population of patients in Rochester, Minnesota, who had to undergo surgery for BPH, 5 mg finasteride administered over a 12 month period provides about 50% of the symptomatic relief attained by surgery (Guess, private communication).

At the conclusion of the 12 month period, patients were enrolled in an open-extension study. After 2 years, preliminary data indicates that the reduction in plasma DHT levels achieved early in the study is well maintained. Prostate volume reduction, which achieved a near maximal response at 6 months, continued slowly for up to 2 years. Serum PSA levels also showed a trend towards continuing decrease, suggesting that the epithelial component of the prostate continues to be affected.

Adverse Effects

There were no significant differences in serious adverse experiences between placebo and finasteride in either study.

Nonserious adverse experiences that occurred with a frequency of more than 2% were sexually related. Decreased libido, decrease in ejaculate volume, and impotence appeared to occur in both finasteride groups at a rate of less than 4% but twice that of the placebo group and these were statistically significantly greater than placebo. However, only one patient discontinued due to a drug-related adverse sexual experience. Preliminary evidence indicates that these sexual dysfunctions are reversible upon drug discontinuation.

Summary and Conclusions

In summary, these studies of over 1800 patients showed that finasteride resulted in improvement in all major parameters tested: prostate volume was reduced, maximum urinary flow rate increased, and urinary symptoms decreased. These beneficial effects have now been well maintained for 2 years (Fig. 2). The long-term use of finasteride has been well tolerated, with no significant toxicity observed in the majority of patients treated.

Data collected thus far demonstrate that the majority of patients exhibit improvement in the symptoms of BPH. It is hypothesized that maintained reduction in prostate volume will alter the natural progression of this disease, but more extensive, long-term, clinical trials will be needed in order to definitely demonstrate this benefit.

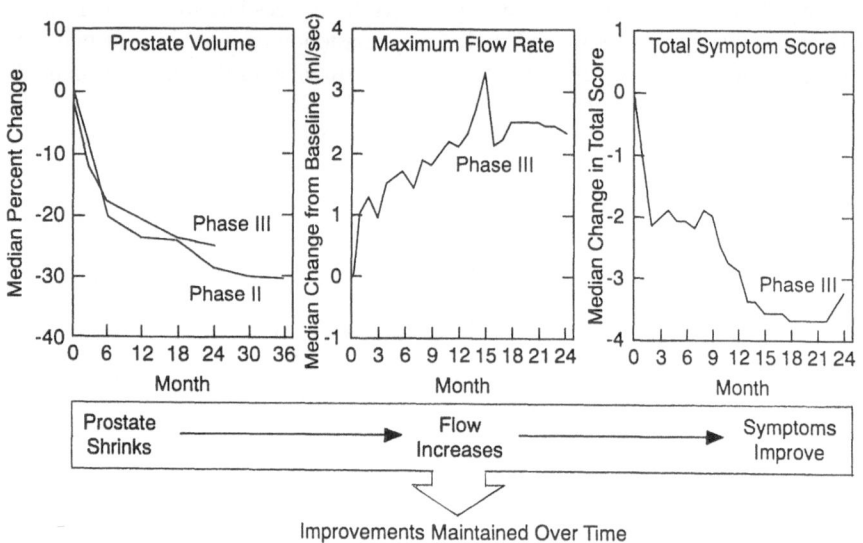

Fig. 2. Summary of long-term effects of finasteride

References

Brooks JR, Berman D, Glitzer MS, Gordon LR, Primka RL, Reynolds GF, Rasmusson GH (1982) Prostate 3:35–44

Brooks JR, Berman C, Garnes D, Giltinan D, Gordon LR, Malatesta PF, Primka RL, Reynolds GF, Rasmusson GH (1986) Prostate 9:65–75

Bruchovsky N, Wilson JD (1968) The intranuclear binding of testosterone and 5α-androstant-17β-01-3-One by rat prostate. J Biol Chem 243:5953

Finasteride Study Group (1991) One year experience in the treatment of BPH with finasteride J Androl 12:372–375

Finasteride Study Group (1992a) Finasteride (MK-906) in the treatment of benign prostatic hyperplasia Prostate (in press)

Finasteride Study Group (1992b) The effect of finasteride in the treatment of men with benign prostatic hyperplasia. N Engl J Med 327:1188–1192

Geller J Franson AV (1989) Effect of MK-906 on prostate tissue androgens and prostate-specific antigen. Seventy-first annual meeting of the Endocrine Society, Seattle, Washington, June Abstr 1640

George FW, Johnson L, Wilson JD (1989) The effect of a 5α-reductase inhibitor on androgen physiology in the immature male rat. Endocrinology 125:2434–2438

Gormley GJ, Rittmaster RS, Gregg H, Lasseter KC, Ferguson D, Stoner E (1989) Dose-response effect of an orally active 5α-reductase inhibitor (MK-906) in man. Seventy-first annual meeting of the Endocrine Society, Seattle, Washington, June Abstr 1225

Imperato-McGinley J (1991) Five alpha-metabolism in finasteride-treated subjects and male pseudo-hermaphrodites with inherited 5α-reductase deficiency: a review. Eur Urol 20(2):78–81

Imperato-McGinley J, Guerrero L, Gautier T, Peterson RE (1974) Steroid 5α-reductase deficiency in man: an inherited form of male pseudohermaphroditism. Science 186:1213–1215

McConnell JD, Wilson JD, George FW, Geller J, Pappas F, Stoner E (1992) Finasteride, an inhibitor of 5α-reductase, suppresses prostatic dihydrotestosterone in men with benign prostatic hyperplasia. J Clin Endocrinol Metab 74:505–508

PROSCAR Study Group (1991) Five alpha-reductase inhibitors in the treatment of benign prostatic hyperplasia (in press)

Rittmaster RS, Stoner E, Thompson DL, Nance D, Lasseter KC (1989) Effect of MK-906, a specific 5α-reductase inhibitor on serum androgens and androgen conjugates in normal men. J Androl 10:259–262

Stoner E (1990) The clinical development of a 5α-reductase inhibitor, finasteride. J Steroid Biochem Mol Biol 37(3):375–378

Stoner E and the Finasteride Study Group (1992) The clinical effects of a 5α-reductase inhibitor, finasteride, on benign prostatic hyperplasia. J Urol 147:1298–1302

Vermeulen A, Giagulli VA, DeSchepper P, Buntinx A, Stoner E (1989) Hormonal effects of an orally active 4-aza steroid inhibitor of 5α-reductase in humans. Prostate 14:45–53

Walsh PC, Madden JD, Harrod JM, Goldstein JL, MacDonald PC, Wilson J (1974) Familial incomplete male pseudohermaphroditism type 2: decreased dihydrotestosterone formation in pseudovaginal perineoscrotal hypospadias. N Engl J Med 291:944–949

Subject Index

Springer-Verlag
and the Environment

We at Springer-Verlag firmly believe that an international science publisher has a special obligation to the environment, and our corporate policies consistently reflect this conviction.

We also expect our business partners – paper mills, printers, packaging manufacturers, etc. – to commit themselves to using environmentally friendly materials and production processes.

The paper in this book is made from low- or no-chlorine pulp and is acid free, in conformance with international standards for paper permanency.